Get Strong Lifelong

Three hours a week
to gain muscle,
lose fat,
and stay healthy
for life.

By Sanjoy Dutta, M.D.

First version: December 2020
Current version: March 2021

Acknowledgements

I dedicate this to my wonderful wife, my two daughters, my parents, my sister, and my friends. All of them give me every reason to live longer and cherish each day.
And to my patients and coworkers, who have helped me grow as both a doctor and a person.

A Request

Promotion and marketing and social media are not my strengths.

So, if you find this book useful, and worth the small investment, please
WRITE A REVIEW on Amazon and recommend it to someone you know.

Would also love to hear your own experience and modifications on
Amazon or Facebook (www.facebook.com/getstronglifelong)

Worksheets are posted on the Facebook site.

Table of Contents

Introduction: Is this book for you?

Do you want to be stronger, healthier, and feel better than ever?
Do you want to be the best physical and emotional version of yourself?
Do you want to prevent diseases that could shorten your life?
Do you want an exercise and diet program that is realistic, practical, and works?
Then this book is for you.

Exercise and a healthy diet help prevent many life shortening diseases such as heart disease, diabetes, dementia, and even cancer. The COVID 19 pandemic has shown us that people with poorer health are even more likely to die from infection. Doctors will always stress the importance of getting healthy, but they don't really tell people how to actually get there. And most exercise and diet programs require an unrealistic amount of time and commitment.

Being healthy, fit, and strong lifelong is easier than you think. This book will tell you what you can do to dramatically improve your health and fitness in a realistic, practical, time efficient, and achievable way. It requires awareness and some willpower, but you can actually be very successful by setting aside just a few hours a week for exercise and making very small adjustments to your diet over time. This book is about choosing the right exercises, improving your understanding of what you eat, carefully measuring your progress, and making micro adjustments to stay successful over a long period of time. Hopefully for life.

If you want to be the healthiest you have been in years and look like it, this book will get you there if:

    1. You can set aside about 3 hours a week (total) for

exercise most weeks.

2. You are willing to increase your awareness about how you eat, and willing to start making some straightforward easy to remember changes for the rest of your life.
3. You are willing to measure your progress and make small adjustments as needed.

This book will provide you with a concrete exercise program and guidelines about how to choose food. But rather than just tell you what to do, the aim of this book is to help you understand how your body physically responds to exercise and food. You can then apply that knowledge to modify and adjust the program provided, to best fit your body, your schedule, and your lifestyle. You DO NOT have to devote unrealistic hours in the gym or follow ridiculous diets with too many rules. That is because the recommendations in this book are based on time tested well-accepted "honest" science and medical knowledge rather than poorly designed science, or "hot off the press" fad science that has not been proven consistently. By understanding how the average human body responds to different types of exercise and food choices, eventually you will learn how your specific body responds to these changes. By closely measuring your progress, you will learn what works best for you. EVENTUALLY YOU MAKE THE RULES. This knowledge will give you the flexibility to design a program that meets your goals not just for a few weeks or months, but for the rest of your life.

The recommendations in this book can be used by any adult, man or woman, trying to get healthier and in better physical shape. However, I do want to admit that there may be some bias towards men's health. Much of my research has been motivated by my own personal interest and experience. I have researched studies on both men and women, and just men, but not studies on just women. There may be hormonal and sex-related differences in the way women respond to diet and exercise which I have not included or researched thoroughly enough. For example, I frequently stress the importance of resistance training and muscle building for long term health. However, I have met many elderly women who seem to be in great physical and mental health without ever having lifted a single weight. Then again, I also know plenty of women who "lift heavy" and can personally swear to the benefits of weight training. I also stress the importance of resistance training, with many exercises targeting the upper body muscles. This probably conforms more to the stereotypical male aesthetic, and not all men and women are interested in gaining a lot of upper body strength. Ultimately, the main purpose of this book is to help you understand what works best for you, so despite the unintended bias towards men, I hope that all genders will still find the recommendations and concepts equally useful and effective.

I am a husband, father, and surgeon in my 50's who has been trying different fitness and diet routines since my 20's. I am also a weight loss surgeon who has spent my career helping people understand how their bodies truly respond to exercise and food, and how to avoid being fooled by the TONS of false information created by people trying to promote their latest fad diet or program or product. There have been periods in my life where I have been able to exercise every day and other periods where I did not exercise for months. Between work and family, it is very difficult to commit to a predictable exercise routine and make progress. After many years of researching different programs, online advice, and the latest exercise and nutrition research, I learned which trainers had the best recommendations, which exercises were the most effective, and which food choices were the most critical. I learned how to make significant progress while still saving time and working around my unpredictable schedule. I feel stronger, more active, and happier in my 50's than I did in my 20's and 30's.

Beware of Short-Term or Extreme Programs
People who are focused on losing fat will often turn to programs and diets that promise significant weight loss in a short amount of time. Weight Watchers, Jenny Craig, Keto, Low Carb, Atkins, Slimfast are examples of diets and programs that may lead to some weight loss over a few months, but are very hard to maintain lifelong. Some of these diets only focus on food and not on exercise and activity. Some of these diets have rules and restrictions that are very hard to follow after a few months, or may be incompatible with other members of the family. Almost all people give up on these programs after a few months, and ultimately gain all or more of their weight back. Yo-yo dieting, which is the term used for losing and gaining weight over and over again, eventually leads to more weight gain and poorer health in the long run.

People who are focused on gaining muscle are usually motivated by a desire to look a certain way, so many of the programs are geared towards achieving that look, rather than gaining muscle to be healthier and more functional. There is usually an unnecessary emphasis on losing total body fat so that the muscles look defined. Once again, these programs require a significant commitment, and are hard to maintain over a lifetime.

The problem with most diets and programs is that they prioritize marketing and business over medical knowledge and science. Sometimes they make programs extremely simple so they are incredibly appealing (i.e. Slimfast), and other times they make the programs intentionally complicated so you become dependent on them (i.e. Weight Watchers points). They claim to have some type of "unique" or "breakthrough" information that will finally get you the results you wish for. Most programs tend to focus on either diet or exercise, but not both. They tend to imply you must follow the program 100% of the time, or it will not work. To make an analogy to finances, many of these diets and programs are like a single stock that promises a big payout, but may ultimately prove to be a big loss. Most investors will tell you that the best long term investment involves diversification and patience.

Long term fitness and health also requires diversification and patience. The best recipe for success involves a combination of eating healthy, maintaining muscle, maintaining cardiovascular fitness, and continually adjusting both diet and exercise when needed. It requires understanding which diet and exercise choices are the most important and effective, and therefore the ones you should try to follow most of the time. It requires understanding which diet and exercise choices may be helpful but less important, and therefore the ones you need to follow only some of the time. And finally it requires you to do your best whenever possible, but not expect yourself to be perfect.

Don't Join the 0.1%

Most of the information on the internet about exercise and diet is overwhelming and confusing. Most of the articles and recommendations are often written by trainers or fitness buffs who seem to be in incredible shape. Many of their recommendations will tell you that you are going to have to be obsessive about food, focused, spend hours in the gym, schedule your life around your workouts, and essentially put the rest of your life on hold. Most of these programs are geared to getting into "superhero" shape. You have to become the stereotypical gym rat and ultra-healthy eater. Why? Because that's what most of these trainers and bodybuilders do. For them, this is their full-time job. Almost all of the programs and regimens and videos and websites are designed by men and women who spend most of their waking hours working out and then trying to somehow make a living out of it. Fitness magazines will convince you that you have to try a new workout regimen every month to keep up. How else would they sell magazines?

If you are like most average people, you have other priorities in life: raising a family, maintaining a home, working probably more than 40 hours a week and perhaps commuting several hours on top of that, paying bills, dealing with illnesses and crises, and hopefully occasionally doing something fun here and there. You are a person with real responsibilities and a real life. So, when you have precious and limited time, your goal should not be to look "shredded" or "ripped" or "buffed" or "jacked." Your goal is to simply look athletic, be stronger, be healthier, and live longer.

If you plot the amount of effort needed vs the actual improvements you make, you can easily guess that the more effort you put, the greater improvements you will see. However, after a certain point, you have to put in a tremendous amount of work into your program to get that "superhero" or "performance athlete look." Your goal should be to get into that zone where you can get as much improvement as possible with as little work as possible. In the graph below, you are going to aim to put just enough work to be in that athletic and strong zone that leads to more functional health and a potentially longer life.

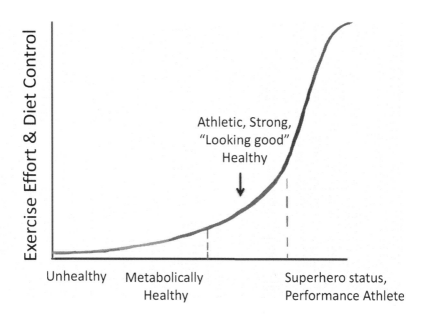

Athletic, Strong, "Looking good" Healthy

Unhealthy   Metabolically
             Healthy

Superhero status,
Performance Athlete

Exercise Effort & Diet Control (y-axis)

Health / Body Type

Join the 12%

In a national study of over 8,700 adults, only about 1 in 8 people (12%) were considered metabolically healthy. (Araujo) They defined metabolically healthy as having a non-obese waist circumference with normal blood pressure, blood glucose, and blood lipids without medications. Good metabolic health is associated with a better quality of life and a longer life.

As we grow older, we hopefully realize that many things we associate with success (money, material wealth, status, recognition, and power) are not as important as life's deeper rewards (love, connection, friendship, meaning and purpose, and appreciation and gratitude). As we grow older, we realize our time here on Earth is limited, and we need to focus on what really matters. Being healthy allows us to experience our life to the fullest and hopefully for as long as possible. There are many aspects of health that are not predictable or fully in our control: accidents, cancer, and many types of diseases can worsen our health dramatically. Yet there are many diseases we can prevent by eating well and being active: obesity, heart disease, high blood pressure, lung disease, joint pains, and injury. So ultimately you need to focus and invest some time on your health so that you can spend more time living the life you want. This program is about how you can make huge improvements in your health, how you feel, and how you look without having to waste excess hours on exercise you don't really need.

To make significant improvements in your fitness and health, you only need to follow some very simple principles:
1. Follow an exercise plan based on consistent medical science and tested studies that you can realistically follow for the rest of your life.
2. Follow a diet plan that is straightforward and based on consistent honest science, that you can realistically follow for the rest of your life.
3. Learn how to continually set micro-goals and make micro-adjustments to your exercise plan and your diet plan. Learn about how your own body responds to different plans.
4. Be realistic and keep perspective. Don't get overly ambitious, but don't give up either.

In practical terms, you need to commit to the following:
1. You should set aside about 3 to 4 hours a week for exercise most weeks. (Spread out over the week as 1 hour 15 min resistance sessions x 2, and 10-30 minute aerobic sessions x 2)
2. You have to be willing to increase your awareness about how you eat, and willing to start making some

straightforward easy to remember changes for the rest of your life.

3. You need to weigh yourself regularly and be willing to measure and record your progress. You need to keep track of your improvement in fitness over time.

You will need the following "materials":

1. Access to free weights in a gym or basic home set up. Weight machines, resistance bands, and body weight exercises (i.e., pull ups, dips, push-ups) are acceptable if free weights are not possible, but free weights are preferable.
2. Some type of aerobic workout set up: running shoes, a bicycle, a stationary bike, etc.
3. A smartphone with a calorie counting app
4. Ideally an activity tracker (Fitbit, watch, etc.) or at least a step counting app on your phone.
5. A scale to weigh yourself at least every other day, and a tape measure to measure your waist.

This book is very short for the following reasons:

1. It is all you really need to know. Books that are longer are just trying to justify their price. Much of the "latest science" promoted in many health books becomes obsolete over time. The problem with the "latest science" is that much of it turns out to be untrue or less clear as more science is done. Unlike technology, when it comes to understanding human biology, newer is not always better. Understanding what has been proven over many years is much more likely to be true.
2. I do not spend too much time describing the actual exercises, because I will let you choose many of the ones that work best for you, and detailed information on any exercise can be found on the internet.

3. You shouldn't be wasting too much time reading or remembering about how to be healthier when you should be living it instead.

Of course, start with caution and common sense

As with any fitness book or program, please consult with your doctor if you have a serious injury or medical condition that can get worse with physical activity or changes in diet. And, as I will mention frequently, start with caution rather than over exuberance. This means that if you have not lifted weights in a long time or ever, always start light. If you have not done aerobic exercise in a long time, start slow. Spend the first few weeks just getting your body used to the idea of exercise. It is always better to start slowly and gradually improve than to push too hard and injure yourself or jeopardize your health

Chap 1. Becoming the Best Version of Yourself

Check your motivation

Before you start this program, you will need to ask yourself what your true motivation is, so you know if this particular program is right for you? Do you want to be healthier, stronger, and be in very good shape compared to most people your age? Are you hoping to improve your ability to experience life and hopefully live longer? If so, then this program will have a lot to offer.

Do you want to spend most of your time with family, loved ones, and at work while still dedicating a small amount of time for yourself to keep yourself healthy and feel great? If so, then this program will have a lot to offer.

Do you want a superhero body? This program can be a very good start, but it's not going to be enough to get you there. As I discussed, getting an extremely muscular low body fat body requires a huge amount of time and commitment. If this is your goal, you really need to ask yourself why is this important to you? Is it for a movie role or a bodybuilding competition? Those are pretty much the only legitimate reasons. Is it to feel better about yourself, or for others to notice you? There are better less superficial ways to achieve that than dedicating hours every day in the gym. And unless you are walking around most of the day with your shirt off, you will probably get more noticed if you dress well. Are you trying to look good for your significant other? Unless they are at the gym with you, you are better off spending time with them rather than away from them working on your body.

Be Realistic

Being realistic is not about lowering expectations, but about keeping them high and redefining them. It is about taking a deep internal look at yourself and asking yourself what you truly want from life, who you really want to be, what is the best use of your time, and how will getting in shape fit into this bigger picture.

Body image in popular culture is unrealistic

Let's look at the recipe for what it takes an actor to get ready for a superhero role. (vice)(melmagazine)(Russo)

First, they start off in pretty good shape, and they were probably born with good genes. Then they start a minimum of 6 months of intense weightlifting workouts several hours a day under the constant supervision of a celebrity trainer. With each rep, the trainer probably pushes the actor by reminding them of the many millions who will be judging them for their shirtless scene. To bulk, they eat meals of plain chicken breast, fish, and red meat six times a day or more, supplemented with several protein shakes. The lucky ones get a "cheat day" once a week. While still training, they shoot most of their movie in costume during their bulked-up phase. Then a few weeks prior to their scheduled shirtless scene they start cutting fat by lowering their calories and spending their days feeling hungry. The day before their scene they stop drinking water. On the day of the scene, they arrive dehydrated and pump up to balloon their body minutes before shooting. That's a lot of sweat, pain, work, and time for only a few seconds of screen time. Bodybuilders similarly spend several years in preparation for their few days of competition: bulking and cutting, spending several hours in the gym daily, eating ridiculously high protein healthy diets, and obsessing constantly about their bodies. When cutting to lower their body fat to unnaturally low levels, they usually feel constantly hungry. The point is that very few people maintain their "ideal look" for a prolonged period of time, much less a lifetime.

Of course, when you go to the gym you will see many young people who are in incredible shape and are not actors or body builders. You will probably see them every time you go there, because they are usually always there. They may often spend several hours a day working out. What motivates them? I'm not sure, but my guess is a bit of insecurity and narcissism. I heard a psychologist once say, "More and more, I find myself treating patients that look like huge men on the outside but turn out to be little boys on the inside."

Normal body fat is okay

Trainers, body builders, models, and gym rats focus on decreasing their overall body fat to almost unnatural amounts, which gives the false impression that body fat is unhealthy and always needs to be reduced as much as possible. Reducing body fat down to 10% or less gives a person the "shredded" and "cut" look of a superhero, and it may give some high-performance athletes an edge (with less weight to carry). Other than improving your shirtless look, trying to look shredded or cut does not really improve your health in a meaningful way and the amount of discipline required to achieve it is difficult for most of us to maintain lifelong. In fact, body fat percentages lower than 5% can be actually dangerous and life threatening.[Padwal] There is also evidence that as we age into our 60's and above, having some extra weight is actually protective against disease and illness.[Pes] There is no strict agreement on what a "healthy" amount of body fat is, and different charts will have very different ranges. There are many men with body fat percentages of 20% or more who are completely healthy and do not need to worry. On the other hand, there may be some men with less than 20% body fat who may need to worry. That is because it is not total body fat, but the fat on the inside of your belly and blood vessels that affects your health. A high waist size carries an increased risk of diabetes, high blood pressure, heart disease, and other diseases. I'll talk about this more in the section on fat.

Becoming stronger, more athletic, and looking good is less effort than you think

Before we delve into the specifics of the program or the workouts, the most important step is to be realistic about individual LIFELONG goals and making a lifelong commitment to attain them.

Here are the MINIMUM ingredients you will need to start this program to make decent progress:

1. Over a period of every 7-9 days, you need to complete the following 4 sessions,
   a. **Weight Workout A:** 1hr 15min resistance training using (preferably) free weights (barbell or dumbbells). Workout A can be split into 2 consecutive days if needed.
   b. **Weight Workout B:** 1hr 15min resistance training using free weights/machines/or body weight exercises. Workout B can be split into 2 consecutive days if needed.
   c. **Aerobic workout 1:** 10-30 min or more of an aerobic workout (can be high intensity)
   d. **Aerobic workout 2:** 10-30 min or more of an aerobic workout (can be high intensity)
   e. Workout A and Workout B need to be spaced at least 48 hours apart. The aerobic workouts can be done at any time. This means a minimum of about 3 hours every 7-9 days TOTAL.

2. You need to understand the total calories you eat, as well as the protein, fat, and carb content in your food. You will need to use a calorie counting app frequently. You will probably need to take protein shakes (or very lean protein) on the days of the resistance workouts and at least the day after.

3. You need to move as much as possible throughout the day. You should preferably use your smartphone or a step counter (Fitbit, smart watch, etc.) to count your daily steps. Most people should eventually aim for an average of 8 - 10,000 steps (or 4-5 miles) a day.

4. You will need to monitor your progress frequently, and make small adjustments towards the direction you want to go. You will focus only the direction you want to go (more muscle OR less fat) but not focus on absolute goals. To measure progress, you will need a scale, and a way to keep track of your exercise.

I will be more specific about the schedule later on, but if you can make the time commitment above, you can easily achieve the following three goals which are the most important elements of your long-term health:

1. **Increased muscle:** Increasing muscle improves your strength and function. It improves your posture and the stability of your spine and joints and prevents injury. Muscle also keeps your metabolism high, allowing you to eat reasonable portions, and of course makes you look athletic, strong, and fit.

2. **Decreased waist size:** If you are carrying extra fat

inside your belly, you need to reduce this to a reasonable size over time. This is the fat that is associated with the most serious health problems. At minimum, you need to make sure you do not gain more fat over time.

3. **Increased cardiovascular fitness:** Over time, your heart and lung function will improve, and you should be able to do more for longer. This will also decrease your risk of both heart and lung disease, which can be a leading cause of death.

As you make progress and get closer to your goals, you will be able to reduce the frequency of the workouts to maintain rather than progress. But I encourage you to at least find a way to set aside as much time as you can for the first several months to make as much improvement as possible as fast as possible. Exercise affects your energy metabolism, oxidative stress, tissue repair, and growth factor response immediately [Contreipois] and you can improve your baseline metabolic health within 6 weeks. [Dunn]

Understanding vs. Doing

Understanding why you need to follow a certain program is helpful, but you will not see any improvements until you actually follow it. On the other hand, when you find yourself following a program but still struggling to make progress or getting confused about what to do, you will have difficulty making effective adjustments unless you understand the science and physiology of your body and the reasoning behind what you do.

Chapter 2 (the science of muscle, fat, and your body) and Chapter 3 (the science of food) are going to be very boring chapters. Most of the information will remind you of high school or college biology class. If you are eager to get started on the program, go to the ends of the chapters and just review the summary.

Chapters 4, 5, and 6 are about the specifics of what you need to do. If you are eager to get started, jump to Chapter 4 and start your routine. Once you have started, however, I strongly recommend you go back to Chapters 2 and 3 so you can build a solid understanding of the science behind the routine. Having this understanding will allow you to maintain your motivation and discipline (especially around food) without having to remember arbitrary rules. It will also help you understand what might be working or not working for you, and how to adjust your exercise and eating to your particular body, metabolism, and schedule. And finally, it will help you understand why many "fast fad" routines may get you better results in a few weeks, but ultimately never work for you in the long run. Ideally over time, if you understand the science of your muscle and your fat, you may come up with a routine that works better for you in the long term than the one I have suggested here.

Citations

1. https://www.vice.com/en_us/article/3kj7d5/models-actors-look-ripped-before-photo-sho
2. https://melmagazine.com/en-us/story/bodybuilders-dehydrate-before-competition-techniques-hugh-jackman-reddit
3. Rossow LM, Fukuda DH, Fahs CA, Loenneke JP, Stout JR. Natural bodybuilding competition preparation and recovery: a 12-month case study. *Int J Sports Physiol Perform*. 2013;8(5):582-592. doi:10.1123/ijspp.8.5.582
4. Araújo J, Cai J, Stevens J. Prevalence of Optimal Metabolic Health in American Adults: National Health and Nutrition Examination Survey 2009-2016. *Metab*

Syndr Relat Disord. 2019;17(1):46-52. doi:10.1089/met.2018.0105

5. Padwal R, Leslie WD, Lix LM, Majumdar SR. Relationship Among Body Fat Percentage, Body Mass Index, and All-Cause Mortality: A Cohort Study. *Ann Intern Med.* 2016;164(8):532-541. doi:10.7326/M15-1181

6. Pes GM, Licheri G, Soro S, et al. Overweight: A Protective Factor against Comorbidity in the Elderly. *Int J Environ Res Public Health.* 2019;16(19):3656. Published 2019 Sep 29. doi:10.3390/ijerph16193656

7. Contrepois K, Wu S, Moneghetti KJ, et al. Molecular Choreography of Acute Exercise. *Cell.* 2020;181(5):1112-1130.e16. doi:10.1016/j.cell.2020.04.043

8. Dunn SL, Siu W, Freund J, Boutcher SH. The effect of a lifestyle intervention on metabolic health in young women. *Diabetes Metab Syndr Obes.* 2014;7:437-444. Published 2014 Sep 19. doi:10.2147/DMSO.S67845

Chap 2. The Science of Muscle, Fat, and Your Body

In this chapter I am going to review how the human body gains muscle and how it loses fat. I will also explain why, unfortunately, it is difficult to do both simultaneously and why you have to focus on one or the other.

Understanding Muscle

Muscle contracts and generates a pulling force.
For the purposes of getting stronger and healthier, we are only concerned with the striated skeletal muscle that helps move your limbs, head, and body. These muscles are made of fibers bundled parallel to each other like wires in a cable. The fibers can contract (pull) together to act as one large muscle. Each fiber is made up of units called sarcomeres. The sarcomeres are lined up one after each other in a row along the entire length of the fiber. The purpose of each sarcomere is to contract and generate a pulling force. Each muscle has a nerve attached to it, and when the nerve sends a signal to contract, all the sarcomeres in all the fibers of the muscle start to contract together. Each sarcomere generates its own tiny pulling force, and because they are all lined up together, attached to each other, and contracting in unison, they act as one single fiber contracting at once. All the fibers contracting at once together act as one large muscle generating a large amount of force. Your nerves can voluntarily control the amount of force your muscle generates by decreasing or increasing the number of fibers activated and recruited. Using every single fiber in a muscle will give you the most strength and force you can get out of that muscle. To get more strength than that, you have to build more fibers.

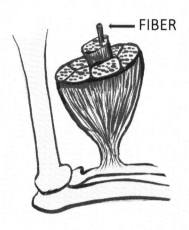

← FIBER

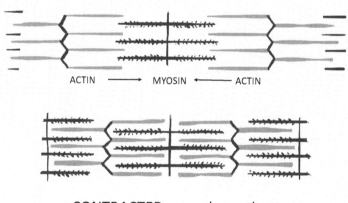

RELAXED = no overlap = long

ACTIN ⟶ MYOSIN ⟵ ACTIN

CONTRACTED = overlap = short

Illustration: Muscle fibers are bundled in parallel to make up the entire muscle. The muscle fiber contracts and shortens by myosin pulling in actin.

How does the sarcomere contract? In each sarcomere there is a network of two long molecules, myosin and actin, that can stick to each other like Velcro when "activated." When the muscle is completely relaxed (as long as possible), the sarcomere is also at its longest, and the myosin and actin have a very small amount of overlap. When the nerve tells the sarcomere to contract (by an influx of calcium into the cell), the myosin is activated, and the myosin starts to pull and stick, pull and stick, and pull and stick to the actin until they are almost completely overlapped and bonded to each other. When the actin and myosin are maximally overlapped, the sarcomere is at its shortest length, and the muscle is as short and contracted as possible. The more the myosin and actin overlap, the stronger the contraction and the force the sarcomere can generate. **This is why your muscle starts out relatively weak when stretched and is strongest when completely contracted.** When the nerve tells the muscle to relax (the calcium concentration goes down) the myosin is deactivated and no longer sticks to actin. At this point the muscle is no longer generating any force.

For the muscle to actually relax and lengthen, a force like gravity or an opposing muscle must pull the opposite way to stretch it out. The myosin can pull the actin in, and let it go, but it cannot push the actin away. Sarcomeres can only generate force when they try to contract, and therefore **muscles can only generate force when contracting (trying to get shorter).** When they deactivate, they relax, and they do not generate any force, and another force outside the muscle must stretch them out. **Muscles cannot generate force when relaxing (and getting longer).** When you do a dumbbell curl, your biceps muscle will shorten to pull your arm and the weight up. When you relax, gravity on the weight will bring your arm down. If you want to bring it down slowly, your bicep

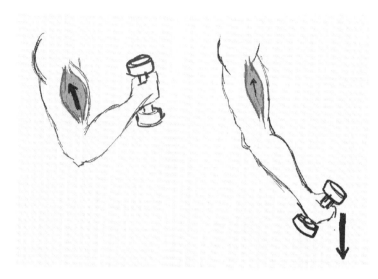

myosin and actin is actually relaxing and contracting extremely quickly against gravity to keep the weight up as gravity brings the weight down. If you were lying on your back (or in a zero-gravity environment) and did a dumbbell curl to your chest, you would have to contract your triceps to get your biceps to stretch back out.

That is why muscles need to work in pairs to create meaningful coordinated movements.

Contraction: Nerve activation → myosin pulls in actin → fiber shortens

Relaxation: Nerve deactivation → myosin lets go of actin → another muscle/force lengthens

Flexion: bending a joint (the flexion muscles contract, the extension muscles relax)

Extension: straightening a joint. (the extension muscles contract, the flexion muscles relax)

The biceps contract and flex your forearm in, and when the biceps relax, the triceps can contract and extend your arms back out. Your hamstrings flex your lower leg in, and your quads extend them back out. Your quads flex your hip (lift your knee up), while your hamstrings and gluteal muscles extend your hip back (lift your knee down).

Muscle fibers come in two forms: slow for sustained activity, and fast for bursts of power.
There are two main types of muscle fibers designed differently for different situations.

Type 1 slow oxidative fibers are designed to burn fuel efficiently over a long time. Because of the biochemical pathways involved, they take longer to generate force, but can generate that force for a longer period of time. They have more mitochondria and ATP (the molecule that stores energy) which function like batteries for the cells, and they can regenerate their ATP very quickly, so they do not require much rest between each movement. They recover quickly. They are good for prolonged sustained activity that does not require a huge burst of strength. Think of them as the Toyota Priuses of muscle fibers.

Type 2 fast muscle fibers use a lot of fuel to generate a lot of power over a short time. When the type 2a fast oxidative muscle runs out of oxygen, the type 2b fast glycolytic can still function for a short time, but fatigue eventually sets in and the fiber has to rest. These fibers take longer (at least 30-60secs) to replenish their energy again. Think of this as your favorite performance car with a V8 engine, horrible gas mileage, and a very small gas tank.

Lucky for you, you have both the ever-practical hybrid and the high-performance car at your disposal. Of course, you might be thinking that the high-performance car is cooler and sexier and that's what we need to work on to be strong. From a strictly superficial perspective, this is partially true. Most men would rather look like a sprinter (more type 2) than a marathon runner (more type1). But don't downplay the importance of your type 1 fibers for health. Without them, you would be exhausted just trying to hold your head up all day. Your daily posture and stability and function depends a lot on healthy type 1 fibers.

Muscle grows in response to trauma
Skeletal muscle can account for 40% of your body mass, and amazingly you may be destroying and replacing up to 1% of your total skeletal muscle every week just due to the wear and tear of being active. Your skeletal muscle is one of the most regenerative tissues in your body (like bone marrow, skin, or liver). If our heart muscle could regenerate with the same ability as our skeletal muscle does, chronic heart disease would not be as life threatening as it currently is.

Trauma (tears, excess activity, inflammation, etc.) damages muscle cells, and as the cells die, they release their contents and chemicals into the tissue. These contents and chemicals signal immune cells to come in and clean the area up within a few hours, and the early immune cells send signals to recruit even more immune cells. Some of these signals also wake up satellite cells in the muscles. Satellite cells are like "baby cells" that cannot do any meaningful work, but can quickly grow up into regular mature muscle cells when asked to and given proper nourishment. These muscle cells can then fuse with your existing muscles cells to replace the damaged portions, and eventually add more muscle than before. Your muscles have lots of satellite cells in wait at all times, ready to grow as needed. Because the signals are spread over a wider area than just the initial injury, satellite cells from all over the "neighborhood" can be recruited to help repair and rebuild.

How long does the process take? The process of inflammation occurs very quickly and continues over the next 36 to 72 hours, by which time most of the damaged tissue is removed. At this point the muscle has recovered enough that it can regain most of its original strength and be stressed (exercised) again. It is unclear how long it takes satellite cells to replace the damaged cells, and eventually increase overall muscle mass. With a consistent exercise program, some studies suggest that noticeable muscle mass can be added within 4 weeks. (Stock)

The other good news is that most people will notice that that even when they stop exercising and start to lose muscle, there is some type of 'muscle memory" that allows them to get back to their previous strength and muscle mass much sooner than the first time around. When you grow muscle, the satellite cells add nuclei to the existing muscle cells to help them grow. Even after the muscles shrink, there is new evidence to suggest that the nuclei still remain, and this allows much faster regrowth the next time around. (Schwartz) This particular finding is too new to make firm recommendations on. However, because the experience of "muscle memory" seems to be common, it is inspiring and motivating to know that the benefit you get from growing muscle is cumulative and lifelong, even if there will be periods in your life when you are not able to exercise or work on muscle growth.

When we try to improve our cardiovascular fitness, we are trying to improve the ability of the heart and lungs to deliver oxygen to our body. Unfortunately, unlike skeletal muscle, your heart muscle does not easily regenerate and form new cells. Instead, the existing cells can grow larger to improve function. This is beneficial to a certain extent, as long as the blood vessels to the heart themselves are wide open. However, if someone has diseased vessels of the heart, the vessels may limit the flow of blood to the heart itself (known as coronary artery disease) and the heart muscle itself will not get enough oxygen as it tries to work harder. If pushed too hard, this can lead to damage or death of some heart muscle, also known as a heart attack. Small amounts of damage to heart muscle can often occur without symptoms. On the other hand, over time new blood vessels can grow in the heart in response to persistent exercise, which is an improvement in heart health and resistance to heart attacks. Therefore, improving heart function and health with regular aerobic exercise is usually greatly beneficial, but it is important to know that you do not have any significant existing heart disease before pushing yourself.

How fast can muscles grow?
There is no clear consensus on how fast weight training can make your muscle grow, but in general it is pretty slow. No matter how much someone works out and eats, the rate of muscle growth is slow because it requires enough damage to promote growth, but not excessive damage that will lead to injury. It is also limited by one's maximum genetic potential for their body to support muscle.   Genetics can account for huge differences among us in how we gain and maintain muscle. When you look at dogs, there are certain breeds that have much more muscle than others, even though they are not doing anything differently than the less muscular dogs. The same differences may also apply to humans. When measured, most sports nutritionists and physicians will quote an average muscle growth of ½ pound to 1 pound a month for athletes and bodybuilders devoting all their time to muscle growth, and not using steroids. There are some individuals who can gain it faster, but they are the exception rather than the rule. As people age, their ability to grow muscle only gets slower. There are also studies that suggest those with heavier and denser bones are

able to grow and support more total muscle than those with lighter bones. Wrist circumference can sometimes be an indicator of how thin or thick your bones might be. Most sports nutritionists and physicians will report that even with regular and intense training, it may take 3 to 5 years for someone to reach their maximum muscle volume.

Big muscles and the Hormonal Effect everywhere.
Multiple studies have shown that heavy weightlifting and other types of high intensity exercises can promote brief rises in testosterone and other hormones in the body. However, the relationship between normal levels of testosterone and muscle growth is complex, so it is not clear if these hormonal changes make a significant difference in your ability to gain muscle or lose fat. Increasing your natural testosterone in small amounts probably does not make it easier to grow muscle. This is the reason why athletes and bodybuilders are tempted to use anabolic steroids, which are designed to act like unnaturally high doses of testosterone. However, a minimum amount of testosterone is needed for muscle growth, and as men age their testosterone levels start to drop. Maintaining muscle mass does seem to help keep the levels higher. Working on the largest muscles are going to lead to much more total muscle mass than smaller muscles, which is why working on your gluteal (butt) muscles, thigh muscles, and back muscles will promote more total muscle growth throughout your body. If your goal is to increase as much muscle mass as possible, then it makes sense to focus on exercises that work on the largest muscle groups, and not waste too much time trying to grow the smaller muscles (like biceps and triceps) that might make your arms look good, but will not improve your overall health, metabolism, strength, and function as much. In other words, if you only have 15 minutes, working on your legs will lead to more muscle growth than working on your arms.

Muscle becomes more important as you grow older

As we grow older, the amount of muscle we have becomes an important predictor of health. A study in 3600 people over age 55 demonstrated that overall muscle mass was a better predictor of living longer than weight. Those in the lowest muscle mass index group were about 80% more likely to die than those in the highest muscle mass index group. (Srikanthan)

Unfortunately, as we grow older, we progressively lose muscle. In a study of men over 65, thigh muscle decreased by 1.2% every year, along with a 1.3% decrease in strength. This 15% decrease in strength over 12 years has more significance than just an increased chance of death. It means decreased ability to walk, get around, drive, open jars, and be independent. (McGregor)

Both resistance training (muscle building) and aerobic training have significant benefits, but as we grow older it becomes even more important to add resistance training in order to prevent muscle loss. As we get older, we become more prone to joint damage and joint injury with extreme aerobic exercise. Proper resistance training can also help prevent injury. On the other hand, it is still important to maintain a moderate amount of aerobic activity to maintain a healthy heart and our overall function. I will review the specifics of aerobic activity in Chap 5.

Your body usually adapts to your rate limiting ability

With every activity, if you do not have an injury, there is ultimately one aspect of your ability and body that will limit you the most and eventually force you to stop or lower your intensity. Think of this as the rate limiting ability. It could be one part of your body that is the weakest. It could be your breathing and feeling out of breath. As you push yourself over time, your body will try to adapt and improve performance by specifically improving your most rate limiting ability. If you are weak but keep trying, you will grow muscle. If you feel short of breath but keep trying your heart and lungs will improve with time. This of course, does not apply to an injury. If you have a sprain or joint that bothers you, pushing yourself will not help and can make your injury worse. You have to wait until the injury is healed before you can push yourself.

Aerobic workouts are limited by cardiovascular fitness rather than muscle size.

An aerobic workout usually involves doing an activity for a long period of time and does not require maximal strength. Examples include running, bicycling, riding a stationary bike, using an elliptical, etc. performed for 30 to 60 minutes or more. Aerobic workouts will require mainly type 1 fibers (the slow, "Prius" fibers). As the muscle fibers use up their large internal store of energy, they need new oxygen delivered to the cells and carbon dioxide to be cleared away. They build up their energy storage relatively quickly and continuously, to keep working with very little or no rest. As the intensity of your aerobic workout increases, the rate limiting ability is usually not your muscle mass or function, but how well your heart and lungs deliver oxygen and clear carbon dioxide through the bloodstream and eventually to your muscles so they can keep going. When you run you do not need to generate that much more force than walking with each movement, but you do have to perform the movements faster. To keep moving, your heart and lungs need to work harder. Over time, your body will adapt to improve your performance in the following ways

1. Your heart and lungs will learn to improve function over time to increase your blood flow and the ability to deliver oxygen and clear carbon dioxide from your tissues. This

is known as cardiovascular fitness.

2. If the force needed with each movement is not that much (i.e., jogging or running on a flat surface), there is no need to significantly increase the number or size of the type 1 muscle fibers. Assuming you currently have enough muscle to walk normally, the muscle that you have is mostly enough to run with moderate intensity. As long as it can get the blood flow it needs, having more muscle is not really going to help. Also the existing muscle can increase their mitochondria to improve their energy storage. They don't need to get bigger, just more energy efficient. This is why long-distance runners can look pretty lean.

3. If more force is required with each movement, and you are not being limited by your cardiovascular fitness, then you will start to make more type 1 fibers to allow you to generate that force. This is why running faster or bicycling up hills will tend to increase the size of the leg muscles over time. However, as the type 1 muscle grows, your cardiovascular fitness will have to improve even further to provide enough blood flow to the now larger muscle.

4. There is really no need to increase the size of type 2 muscle fibers, since they are not as "fuel efficient" as the type 1 fibers, can only help for a short amount of time (minutes), and would only add extra weight to your body.

Strength workouts are limited by your muscle function and size.

Strength workouts involve activities that require you to use more force than aerobic workouts. These can include using the same aerobic machines as above, but with the resistance set so high you can only do it for less than a minute or two. Strength workouts can include bands or machines with high resistance (weight machines, pulleys, bands, etc.), exercises that require you to lift your body weight (pull ups, dips, push-ups, etc.) and free weight exercises (dumbbells, barbells, etc.). These exercises are usually performed in short bursts with periods of rest in between. These activities are mostly limited by your muscle mass and how much force they can generate. Improving your cardiovascular fitness and improving your blood flow to the muscle will not really improve your strength, since the movement really depends on energy that was already stored in the muscle. Theoretically, if you held your breath while lifting a heavy weight 6 to 8 times, it should not make much of a difference in your strength. The main reason you breathe during the exercise is to stay relaxed, keep focused, and deliver oxygen to your brain. As you try to lift a heavy weight you will recruit as much muscle fiber as possible to perform the task. All the muscle fibers will be recruited, but once the type 2 fibers (fast, "V8 engine") run out of energy there won't be enough strength to continue the activity and it will take some time for the muscles to recharge their battery (mitochondria) before trying again. "The burn" you feel is lactic acid building up in the muscle, which is a by-product of your muscle using energy. Your limiting ability is not energy delivery, but the amount of muscle you have to generate force. The more muscle you have, the more force you can generate. This muscle will be using energy that was already stored in it. If you are doing an exercise that involves several different muscles, you will put the most stress on the muscle that is the weakest and limiting you the most. Therefore, that is the most likely to increase over time. This is a good thing. For example, if you start doing a bench press and start to notice that your arms are more tired than your chest, most of your muscle growth will occur in your arms first.

As you continue to lift heavy weights, your body will adapt in the following ways

1. Your existing muscle will improve its ability to generate force by improving the way its fibers work together. It can increase mitochondria and store more energy.
2. In response to small tears and damage from each workout, the satellite cells will help the muscle grow more cells and fibers, so that over time you can generate more and more force.
3. Cardiovascular fitness will also improve a little bit to improve blood flow to the larger energy spending muscle, but most of the energy comes from energy that is already stored in the muscle before you start the exercise.

Aerobic and Strength Workouts: a recap

1. With aerobic workouts your body will adapt by improving energy efficiency and delivery.
2. With resistance and weight workouts your body will adapt by increasing muscle strength and mass.

Of course, many exercises have a component of both, but the good news is that with enough exercise, your body will try to improve your performance over time. Unfortunately, the opposite is true as well. When you stop being active, your cardiovascular fitness declines. You start to lose muscle again because all types of muscle need a large amount of energy to live and function, and are relatively "expensive" if not being used. Muscle "charges a lot of rent" to hang around. Elderly people who are bedridden for even a few days in the hospital can quickly lose the strength to even stand up. (English)

On the other hand, as I mentioned before, the good news is there is some type of 'muscle memory" that allows us to get back our previous strength and muscle mass much sooner than the first time around. So, increasing your muscle mass now will have lifelong benefits even if you have setbacks or short periods of inactivity and muscle loss. And of course, every day that you dedicate to aerobic activity and cardiovascular fitness makes you less likely to develop diseases like hypertension, diabetes, and heart disease.

Another piece of good news is that even people who have a hard time improving with aerobic activity seem to improve when they switch to resistance training, and vice versa. In a recent study, twins spent three months biking three times a week, and then another three months weightlifting three times a week. (Marsh) As expected for most people, biking improved endurance more than leg strength, while resistance training improved leg strength more than endurance. There were a few people who responded poorly to one type of exercise, but luckily seemed to respond well to the other. So, the good news is that most people respond to both types of exercise, and everyone should respond to at least one type. Which is why I recommend starting with a program that incorporates both aerobic and resistance training. The study did not look into how these people responded to a combined program. Another interesting finding of the study was that identical twins did not seem to respond any more "identically" than the fraternal twins. This suggests that genetics had less influence than anticipated. It is possible that environment, prior health, and lifestyle can also help determine how well our bodies respond to different types of exercise. This implies that in the long term, as we improve our endurance and strength, we may be able to also improve our ability to respond to exercise. At the same time, we must be willing to adjust our exercise routines to give us the maximal improvement for our effort.

Understanding Fat

Fat has function

Fat cells can be found in almost all parts of our body: under our skin, around our intestines, in our liver, around our heart and blood vessels, and speckled in our muscles. In addition to insulating the body, fat is mainly a tissue for energy storage. It can be broken down to provide energy to the body when food is no longer available. One pound of fat can provide approximately 3500 calories of energy, which is more than most people need to survive two to three days without food. If you eat more food than you use, it makes complete sense for the body to store that extra energy in the form of fat. Think of fat as a savings account or "rainy day fund" for all the energy you ate and never used but is at your disposal if you ever need it. In the days when food and energy were scarce, it made sense for your body to have this energy 'savings account". In addition, fat tissue does very little work compared to other tissues and needs very little energy to live. Because the "fees" to maintain this savings account are so low, fat tends to stick around for a long, long time. Keeping fat is cheap. This is the opposite of muscle, which requires a lot of energy to maintain, and is "expensive" to keep around.

From an evolutionary perspective, there may be good reasons human beings are meant to form fat.
1. It allows people to survive long periods of famine
2. It gives people reserve to make long distance journeys and explore new lands without knowing when food will be available right away
3. It helps keep us warm and survive colder temperatures.

As long as we live in an environment of abundance, it makes complete sense for the body to make more fat. To be honest, this "thrifty gene hypothesis" may not fully explain the epidemic of obesity in our population, but it does help us understand why our body has more natural mechanisms to gain fat rather than lose it.

In addition to energy, fat also provides insulation. The function of fat in the brain and around nerves is very different but is not important for this discussion. A special type of fat called brown fat can actually help you burn calories but is usually a tiny fraction of your total fat. There may be some people lucky to be born with more brown fat than others. For most of us, though, trying to lose fat means focusing on trying to lose the fat that is being used as energy storage.

The bad news: Metabolic adaptation makes losing fat difficult.

So, the great news is that your body can respond to activity by improving your cardiovascular fitness or your muscle. Your body adapts to the stress of the activity.

Unfortunately, that same activity does not signal your body to lose fat.

There is absolutely no reason for your body to lose fat unless it is starving, and even in that case, it does not want to. (ochner)

Here is a depressing example of why it is so difficult to lose fat: Let's assume Martin, who is overweight at 249lbs, eats 2100 calories a day because that is what he heard the average American diet should be. Unfortunately, because he has a long commute and a desk job, he is not very active, and only burns about 1600 calories a day to stay alive (his basal metabolism). The extra 500 calories of food over 7 days adds up to 3500 calories, or one pound of fat at the end of the week. When Martin overeats, there are no warnings to his body to stop, because as we noted, the human body views fat formation as a good thing.

Martin suddenly becomes aware of his weight as the scale hits 250lbs for the first time and he decides to go on a crash diet. He downloads a calorie counting app and decides to drop down to about 1100 calories a day but does not become more active. If we do the math, we would assume that with this diet he should be able to lose 500 calories a day (1600 calories for his basal metabolism - 1100 calories eaten = 500 calories needed from fat) and therefore lose his extra pound of fat in one week. Unfortunately, this is not the case.

Although his body didn't mind storing the extra calories when he ate too much, his body will feel something is terribly wrong when he eats too little. The body becomes concerned that there may not be enough food in the environment, and that Martin is living in a land of food scarcity. To prevent him from starving to death, Martin's body will "metabolically adapt" by lowering his basal metabolism. This is called "adaptive thermogenesis". It may drop down to 1400, or even 1200 calories instead. So, at a 1200 calorie per day basal metabolism on a 1100 calorie a day diet, he will only be depleting 100 calories of his fat every day, and it will now take 35 days to lose that same pound.
It took one week to gain a pound of fat but will take one month to lose it!!!
Martin realizes his crash diet is not working, and decides to add exercise, and burns an extra 400 calories a day on the treadmill. The good news is that if Martin can continue to exercise and stick to his 1100 calorie a day diet and 400 calorie a day exercise plan, he will lose fat. The hard part is that calorie restriction and the exercise will both increase glucocorticoids and other hunger hormones that will increase hunger and the ability to store fat, making his routine harder and harder to stick to.

As you see, the body has many built in evolutionary

mechanisms to either preserve or gain weight, but has no natural mechanisms to help you lose fat. You have been growing your entire life, and the body views that as a positive direction. There is no "natural" or biologic mechanism that realizes when your extra fat may be actually harming you, and helps you lose fat. Because you cannot let your body "guide" you naturally, if you want to lose fat, you must take control of your diet and activity consciously and deliberately.

Abdominal fat matters more than any other type.

BMI and total body fat percentage are not very good indicators of the fat that you need to get rid of.

BMI refers to body mass index, which is your weight (in kilograms) over your height squared (in meters^2). If you do not know your BMI, use any BMI calculator on the internet. Under 18 is considered anorexic (unhealthy low weight), 18 to 25 is considered a normal range, 25 to 30 is considered overweight, 30 to 40 is considered obese, and over 40 is considered morbidly obese. When applied across a huge population, these categories can indicate an increased risk of disease. Populations who are obese and morbidly obese can have statistically higher chances of high blood pressure, heart attack, diabetes, sleep apnea and other medical problems. However, you cannot always apply this BMI risk to an individual person. People with a lot of muscle will have higher BMI's but will not have any increased risk. Many wrestlers and body builders like the Rock or Arnold Schwarzenegger (in his prime) had BMI's greater than 30, but they were not obese or unhealthy. There are some people who can carry a lot of extra fat in the morbidly obese range without developing medical problems. On the other hand, there are some people in the overweight range who develop medical problems with just a small amount of extra fat.

Trainers and body builders aiming for that extremely muscular defined appearance put a lot of emphasis on total body fat percentage. They often talk about trying to get to less than 10% body fat, which is why they ultimately promote a routine of bulking and cutting. During bulking, they gain more muscle than they need, and gain some fat along with it. During cutting, they hope to lose more fat than muscle, but realize that they will still lose some muscle and strength. And they know they cannot stay at extremely low body fat percentages of 6-8% permanently. Bulking and cutting is all about trying to achieve the muscular super low body fat look for a short amount of time, but there is absolutely no health benefit to having an abnormally low body fat percentage. And it is extremely difficult to maintain for a long period of time.

The fat you DO need to reduce is the fat inside your abdomen, around the internal organs of your belly. This is not the fat that is under your skin or even the fat on your waist that you can pinch with your fingers, which is the fat that is around your abdomen. Under that fat is another layer of muscle and connective tissue (fascia) that gives your abdomen strength and keeps all your abdominal organs inside. Your abdominal organs include organs like the liver, spleen, pancreas, and intestines. Your liver can be filled with a large amount of fat. The blood vessels to your intestines are surrounded by fat, and there is also an apron of fat called the omentum that blankets the intestine. This fat inside the abdomen is clearly associated with a higher risk of diseases such as diabetes, heart disease, high blood pressure, heartburn, and difficulty breathing. This is why trying to reduce your overall waist size is more important to your health than trying to lose your total body fat percentage.

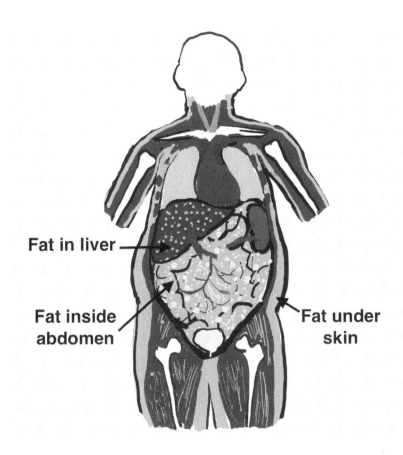

Fat in liver

Fat inside abdomen

Fat under skin

Numerous studies demonstrate that for both men and women, higher waist sizes are associated with significantly higher rates of medical problems such as diabetes and heart disease and early death. Waist size is always measured at the belly button, so it is the measurement around your midsection, not your pant size. Your pant size is your hip circumference. The studies often have different cutoffs so it is hard to make an absolute rule, but in general we can expect that men with waist sizes of 45 have about twice the risk of death compared to men with smaller waists (35 inches or less). For women, a waist size of 42 inches has twice the risk of death compared to a waist size of 29.5 inches or less. And if the risk of death is twice as high, the risk of diabetes, heart disease, and cancer will be even higher. [Jacobs]

Similar studies seem to suggest that the risk of heart disease and diabetes starts to increase after 40 inches for men, and 35 inches for women.[Cerhan, Despres]

The bad news is that you CANNOT SPOT REDUCE fat. Doing aerobic exercise with your arms will not make you lose fat in your arms. Doing lots of crunches may promote muscle growth but will not reduce fat around your belly. When you burn energy, your body determines where it will burn the fat first. It could be any part of your body. Luckily, for most people, it is usually the fat inside the abdomen and in your liver that you usually burn first. This means you won't lose your love handles easily but you usually will decrease your overall waist size as you try.

Summary: Muscle and Fat and How Your Body Adapts to Exercise

1. Your body tries to adapt to your rate limiting ability (as long as you do not have an injury). With aerobic exercise, your body will try to improve cardiovascular fitness (oxygen and energy delivery) and type 1 (slow) muscle fibers. With weightlifting and resistance training, your body will try to increase its muscle mass and type 2 (fast) fibers. You will most likely stress and increase the muscle that is the weakest for a particular exercise.

2. Muscle is expensive because it requires a lot of energy to maintain. If your body truly needs more muscle (because you are stressing it and damaging it) and you are eating enough protein to make more muscle, the body will adapt by adding more muscle to your normal (genetically and hormonally determined) amount. If you don't continue to push your muscle to work, however, you can quickly lose it again. Luckily, there is some

"muscle memory" when you start working out again.

3. Increasing your bigger muscles will help your smaller muscles grow, but not the other way around.

4. Your body will make some fat whenever you eat a little extra. Fat is cheap to maintain and likes to stick around. Even if the extra fat is contributing to medical problems (like diabetes, sleep apnea, high blood pressure, etc.) your body does not care. Your body thinks extra fat is a good thing.

5. When you try to lose fat by eating much less, "adaptive thermogenesis" and other body mechanisms fight against you, lowering your metabolism and increasing your hunger. Losing fat requires deliberate, conscious, and measured effort.

6. You CAN increase muscle in a specific area.

7. You CANNOT reduce fat in a specific area.

Citations

1. Stock MS, Mota JA, DeFranco RN, et al. The time course of short-term hypertrophy in the absence of eccentric muscle damage. *Eur J Appl Physiol.* 2017;117(5):989-1004. doi:10.1007/s00421-017-3587-z

2. Schwartz LM. Skeletal Muscles Do Not Undergo Apoptosis During Either Atrophy or Programmed Cell Death-Revisiting the Myonuclear Domain Hypothesis. *Front Physiol.* 2019;9:1887. Published 2019 Jan 25. doi:10.3389/fphys.2018.01887

3. Srikanthan P, Karlamangla AS. Muscle mass index as a predictor of longevity in older adults. *Am J Med.* 2014;127(6):547-553. doi:10.1016/j.amjmed.2014.02.007

4. McGregor RA, Cameron-Smith D, Poppitt SD. It is not just muscle mass: a review of muscle quality,

composition and metabolism during ageing as determinants of muscle function and mobility in later life. *Longev Healthspan*. 2014;3(1):9. Published 2014 Dec 1. doi:10.1186/2046-2395-3-9

5. English KL, Paddon-Jones D. Protecting muscle mass and function in older adults during bed rest. *Curr Opin Clin Nutr Metab Care*. 2010;13(1):34-39. doi:10.1097/MCO.0b013e328333aa66

6. Marsh CE, Thomas HJ, Naylor LH, Scurrah KJ, Green DJ. Fitness and strength responses to distinct exercise modes in twins: Studies of Twin Responses to Understand Exercise as a THerapy (STRUETH) study [published online ahead of print, 2020 Jun 22]. *J Physiol*. 2020;10.1113/JP280048. doi:10.1113/JP280048

7. Ochner CN, Barrios DM, Lee CD, Pi-Sunyer FX. Biological mechanisms that promote weight regain following weight loss in obese humans. *Physiol Behav*. 2013;120:106-113. doi:10.1016/j.physbeh.2013.07.009

8. Jacobs EJ, Newton CC, Wang Y, et al. Waist circumference and all-cause mortality in a large US cohort. *Arch Intern Med*. 2010;170(15):1293-1301. doi:10.1001/archinternmed.2010.201

9. Cerhan JR, Moore SC, Jacobs EJ, et al. A pooled analysis of waist circumference and mortality in 650,000 adults. *Mayo Clin Proc*. 2014;89(3):335-345. doi:10.1016/j.mayocp.2013.11.011

10. Després JP. Waist circumference as a vital sign in cardiology 20 years after its initial publication in the American Journal of Cardiology. *Am J Cardiol*. 2014;114(2):320-323. doi:10.1016/j.amjcard.2014.04.043

Other References

1. Textbook of Medical Physiology 12th Ed. Guyton and Hall. Unit II Membrane physiology, nerve, and muscle. Chap 6. Contraction of Skeletal muscle. C.2011
2. Purves D, Augustine GJ, Fitzpatrick D, et al., editors. The Regulation of Muscle Force. Neuroscience. 2nd edition.Sunderland (MA): Sinauer Associates; 2001.
3. www.khanacademy.org/science/health-and-medicine/human-anatomy-and-physiology/introduction-to-muscles/v/type-1-and-2-muscle-fibers
4. https://www.health.harvard.edu/staying-healthy/exercise-and-aging-can-you-walk-away-from-father-time
5. Bhasin S, Apovian CM, Travison TG, et al. Effect of Protein Intake on Lean Body Mass in Functionally Limited Older Men: A Randomized Clinical Trial. *JAMA Intern Med.* 2018;178(4):530-541. doi:10.1001/jamainternmed.2018.0008
6. Fothergill E, Guo J, Howard L, et al. Persistent metabolic adaptation 6 years after "The Biggest Loser" competition. *Obesity (Silver Spring).* 2016;24(8):1612-1619. doi:10.1002/oby.21538
7. Karalaki M, Fili S, Philippou A, Koutsilieris M. Muscle regeneration: cellular and molecular events. *In Vivo.* 2009;23(5):779-796.
8. Lee JJ, Pedley A, Hoffmann U, Massaro JM, Fox CS. Association of Changes in Abdominal Fat Quantity and Quality With Incident Cardiovascular Disease Risk Factors. *J Am Coll Cardiol.* 2016;68(14):1509-1521. doi:10.1016/j.jacc.2016.06.067
9. Shadrin IY, Khodabukus A, Bursac N. Striated muscle function, regeneration, and repair. *Cell Mol Life Sci.* 2016;73(22):4175-4202. doi:10.1007/s00018-016-

2285-z

10. Yang W, Hu P. Skeletal muscle regeneration is modulated by inflammation. *J Orthop Translat.* 2018;13:25-32. Published 2018 Feb 7. doi:10.1016/j.jot.2018.01.002

Chap 3. The Science of Food

Food is Chemistry

What is food? Food is any substance we can digest (break down) and get energy from. Humans and most animals get their energy from only three types of food molecules: carbohydrates, fats, and protein.

Carbohydrates

Carbon, Hydrogen, and Oxygen are bonded in hexagon or pentagon pattern to make molecules of sugar. Sugar is the basic unit or building block for all carbohydrates. Sugars like glucose, or fructose can stand alone (monosaccharides). Or they can come in pairs (disaccharide). The most common disaccharide we eat is sucrose (table sugar), made of one glucose and one fructose (shown below). Sugars are very easy to break down and build up again chemically. Sugars can also be combined into long chains, known as polysaccharides. Starch is an example of a polysaccharide made from long glucose chains.

Fats

Carbon, Hydrogen, and Oxygen can be bonded in a different way to make glycerol and chains of fatty acids. The building blocks of glycerol and fatty acids combine together to make different types of fat. Fats are also relatively easy to break down or build up again in our bodies.

$$H-\underset{\underset{H}{|}}{\overset{\overset{H}{|}}{C}}-\underset{\underset{H}{|}}{\overset{\overset{H}{|}}{C}}-\underset{\underset{H}{|}}{\overset{\overset{H}{|}}{C}}-\underset{\underset{H}{|}}{\overset{\overset{H}{|}}{C}}-\underset{\underset{H}{|}}{\overset{\overset{H}{|}}{C}}-\overset{\overset{O}{\|}}{C}-OH$$

$$H-\underset{\underset{H}{|}}{\overset{\overset{H}{|}}{C}}-\underset{\underset{H}{|}}{\overset{\overset{H}{|}}{C}}-\overset{\overset{H}{|}}{C}\equiv C-\underset{\underset{H}{|}}{\overset{\overset{H}{|}}{C}}-\overset{\overset{O}{\|}}{C}-OH$$

$$H-C\equiv C=C=C\equiv C-\overset{\overset{O}{\|}}{C}-OH$$

Protein

Carbon, Hydrogen, Oxygen, and Nitrogen are bonded together in a specific pattern to make molecules called amino acids. Notice that protein is the only compound to also have Nitrogen. There are only 20 amino acids in humans, and they can be linked together in billions of ways to create billions of different proteins. Humans can put together carbon, hydrogen, oxygen, and nitrogen to make amino acids, and then put these together to make proteins. Making amino acids and protein is much more complicated chemically than making carbohydrates or fat. In addition, we only have the chemistry skills to build 11 of the 20 amino acids. There are 9 amino acids that we cannot make, and we must consume them from food in order to have enough supply to build the many proteins we need to live. The molecules below are some examples of amino acids, but hundreds and thousands of amino acids will connect to make actual proteins. That is why breaking down and building protein takes a LOT more work.

The Energy in Food: Where is it?

You probably know that we eat food to obtain energy, but do you know where in the food is the energy actually found?

The energy in food is found within the molecular (covalent) bonds between the carbon, hydrogen, oxygen, and nitrogen atoms. In the diagrams above, the bonds are represented by all the lines between the molecules. Our body breaks down food and eventually breaks some of the bonds between molecules and atoms, which releases energy. The process of breaking down food is called digestion. The energy from broken bonds is quickly captured to create new bonds in energy transfer molecules (primarily ATP), that then store the energy until they are used for the billions of chemical reactions throughout your body. This is how food allows you to live. The transfer molecules can also deliver energy to the parts of your body that need to make muscle (primarily protein), fat, or carbohydrates.

So, in other words, your body knows how to break down proteins, carbs, and fats (from outside the body) in order to get energy, and then can use this energy to make its own proteins, carbs, and fats.

Our bodies do not digest proteins, carbs, and fats equally. It turns out that when you eat protein, you may use up 30% of the energy just trying to break down the protein molecules themselves, so you only get 70% of the energy listed on the food label. In contrast, digesting fat may take very little energy, and you tend to get 98% of the energy listed on the food label. We will talk about this more in the section on digestion. If you look at the molecules, you can guess that a more complicated molecule takes more work to break down and build again.

On a side note, all animals get their energy from food. All food is either other animals or plants. As you follow the food chain, ultimately all the energy originally comes from plants alone, which create food molecules using the energy of sunlight. This means that ultimately the energy of all living organisms on planet earth comes from the sun. The energy you use to read this book or walk across the room is energy that once came from the sun. All life on earth is solar powered.

Fiber

Fiber (roughage, bulk) is a type of carbohydrate that you CANNOT digest or break down for energy. So technically fiber is not a food. Fiber is important for your digestive system because it helps you maintain healthy bacteria in your large intestine and gives substance to healthy bowel movements. Fiber can also help you feel full without any calories being absorbed into your body. To be completely honest, certain types of fibers called soluble fibers are broken down by bacteria. The by-products of this breakdown include fatty acids that you do actually absorb into your body. But for the most part this is a very small contribution to the calories you get from food.

Vitamins and Minerals

Vitamins (A, B1, B6, B12, C, D, E, K, etc.) are molecules and minerals (Iron, Calcium, Zinc, Copper, etc.) are elements that you need to complete certain enzymes or parts of your body. For example, your blood cells need iron to help make hemoglobin, and your body needs calcium to help make bones. You do not break down or digest vitamins or minerals. So technically they are not food, because you do not derive energy from them. Instead, you absorb them from your food and into your body, to be used as needed. Think of them as "special pieces" you need to help you create certain types of proteins or keep specific body parts functioning.

Calories: A measurement of energy

We eat food to obtain energy. Calories are a unit of energy. We use calories to measure the amount of energy in food, a chemical reaction, or any activity. The more calories, the more energy.

How many calories should you eat each day? It all depends. If you do not want to gain or lose weight, you need to eat just enough calories to give you the energy you need to do whatever you need to do. If you have less, you won't have enough energy to finish your day, and you'll have to tap into energy stores in your body. If you have more, you will store the extra energy somewhere in your body. Bodybuilders and actors getting big for their roles may consume 4000-6000 calories a day, mostly protein. Olympic athletes like Michael Phelps supposedly needed 8-10,000 calories a day when training. The average "recommended" American diet is supposedly 2000 to 2500 calories a day, but this is not really based on good science. In reality, most average sized adults would do fine eating much less (about 1200 to 1600calories a day). They might be a bit skinnier and feel hungry throughout the day, but they also may actually live longer. (Mattison, Wilcox)

So, let's take a look at the amount of calories in fat, muscle, and carbohydrates.

	calories/gram	calories/pound (estimated)
protein	4	1800
carbs	4	1800
fat	9	4100*

*Wait, didn't we mention that 1 lb. of fat is about 3500 calories? In actuality, 1 lb. of pure fat (like a stick of butter) is about 4100 calories. Human body fat is about 70-90% fat and the rest is water and proteins and connective tissue. So, a pound of human fat is estimated to be about 3500 cals. Of course, it can vary greatly among individuals and even in different parts of the body.

Similarly, muscle is not made out of pure protein, and a pound of human muscle may yield only about 700 calories because so much of it is water and blood vessels and connective tissue.

Hunger and the availability of food.

Hunger is a drive that originates in the hypothalamus in the brain. There may be hormones from other parts of the body (the stomach, intestine, pancreas, fat, etc.) that may influence our hunger, but ultimately all hunger originates from this center in the brain.

Why are we born with hunger?

Let's take two people: one who NEVER gets hungry and one who is ALWAYS hungry and put them on a deserted tropical island. Which of these two people is more likely to survive? For some reason, even though I think the answer is obvious, when I ask this question many people think the person who is never hungry will survive. Maybe they think the hungry person will be so miserable they will not survive, or they need to eat more because they are hungrier. Maybe they think that a person who isn't hungry doesn't need to eat, which of course is not true. Every person MUST eat to get a certain amount of energy in order to live. In this case, the person who is never hungry is more likely to sit by the beach and enjoy the view a few days until they realize they are suddenly very dehydrated and weak. When they make the rational decision to look for food, it may be too late. Meanwhile the person who is always hungry will start looking for food and water right away. They will do whatever it takes: find water and try to purify it, find fruits, set traps, think about fishing, etc. Even though feeling hungry all the time may be hard on them mentally, their hunger will push them to actually find water and food, and therefore survive.

From an evolutionary perspective, if humans are living in a world where food is scarce, it makes sense to have a high hunger drive. This is the same food scarce evolutionary environment that selected the "adaptive thermogenesis" we talked about earlier: the body's ability to create and hold onto as much fat as possible in order to survive long stretches of starvation and famine.

And that is the biggest problem in our modern world: food is no longer scarce. In 1890, 90% of the world's population lived in extreme poverty and could barely eat, and today only 10% of the world's population lives in extreme poverty. [Pinker] The great majority of human beings on this planet, for the first time in history, can eat whenever they want. Hunger is a reminder to look for food. People used to walk around for hours, sometimes days, hungry and looking for food. Now they spend a few minutes. Hunger is such a strong drive that it has pushed human beings to use their ingenuity to create ways to get food faster and cheaper and more abundantly. And because we have succeeded, and evolution has not adapted to this new normal, we are now victims of our own success.

In today's society, feeling hungry probably leads to eating more than we really need to. Some of us find ways to burn that extra energy off, while many of us simply store it as fat. If hunger were the only reason we ate, it would be bad enough. But unfortunately, we often eat for reasons that have nothing to do with hunger. Think about all the times you may have eaten for any of the following reasons, and check the box if you have.

- ❏ being bored. (i.e., nothing to do, raid the cupboard or refrigerator to munch on something)
- ❏ being social (i.e., a party, BBQ, celebration dinner)
- ❏ for entertainment (i.e., movie popcorn or candy, food at a sporting event or show)
- ❏ for reward (i.e., an ice cream with your kids, a drink after a hard day's work)
- ❏ to soothe emotions, stress, fatigue, or anxiety (i.e., a bowl of ice cream or a drink help dull uncomfortable emotions)
- ❏ by chance. The food happened to be there. (i.e., coworkers bring in food, somebody else is eating a snack)
- ❏ for cravings and pleasure. Is a craving the same as hunger, or is it a desire or thought for a food you think will bring you pleasure?

The evolutionary strength of hunger, the easy availability of food, and a tendency to eat even when not hungry all contribute to us eating more than we biologically need to.

How do I eat? Digestion determines the actual calories you get

Your digestive system starts with your mouth and then your stomach, which breaks down food mechanically and chemically. After your food leaves the stomach and travels through the intestine, food is broken down chemically with the help of bile and enzymes secreted by the liver and pancreas. The molecules of food (sugars, fatty acids, and amino acids), vitamins, and minerals are absorbed by the intestine and into the bloodstream.

When you look at a food label for the amount of calories in a food, these numbers represent the most calories you could get from that food, but not necessarily the net calories your body will actually absorb. This is because the calories reported on the label are based on how food is burned in a chamber in the lab. But your body does not burn food in the same way. A good example of this is hay. If you purchase hay for your horse or cow, you may buy hay that has about 800 calories per pound. When the cow eats this hay, they actually do not even get energy from the hay. The hay is fermented and used to grow bacteria, which is where the cow gets its nutrients. If you eat hay, you will not get any calories.

Sugars and fats do not take much work to digest. (Dunn) This means that most of the calories you see on the label will be absorbed. Proteins are the hardest type of food to digest. 100 "label" calories of proteins may only lead to a net gain of 70 calories into your body. (Mattes)

	"Label" calories	"Net Digested" calories
fat	100 (9 cal/ gram)	97-100
sugar	100 (4 cal/ gram)	90 - 95 95 - 99 for sugar drinks
protein	100 (4 cal/ gram)	65 - 80
alcohol	100 (7 cal / gram)	99-100
Insoluble fiber	100 (4 cal / gram)	0

When you use calorie counting apps or look at food labels, you will only get values of the "label" calories. You will have to use your understanding of the chart above to get a rough estimate of how many of those label calories are actually getting into your body.

Ultimately it is the net digested calories that will determine how well you gain muscle or lose fat.

Carbohydrates and the Glycemic Index

When it comes to carbohydrates, digestion depends on how much the carbohydrate acts like a sugar. This is measured by their glycemic index. Simple sugars have a high glycemic index, which means they are absorbed very quickly. A label with 100 calories for a high glycemic food may give you 95 to 100 calories, and most of these calories are absorbed very quickly. This can cause hormonal highs and lows that can often worsen hunger. White rice, white bread, bagels, instant oatmeal, potatoes, and cornflakes are examples of high glycemic foods that are easily and quickly absorbed.

Carbohydrates like whole grain wheat bread, steel cut oats, sweet potatoes, and brown rice have a low glycemic index. They take more work and longer to break down than simple sugars.

They do not cause hormonal highs and lows, and are less likely to lead to hunger. A label with 100 calories for a low glycemic food may give you only 90 calories. The low glycemic food will take longer to digest, and therefore satisfy your hunger better. As a side note, many breads will say "whole grain added" which just means a small portion of the bread is actually whole grain. Look for breads that say "100% whole grain."

Processed Foods

There are also some studies that suggest processed foods have a much higher percentage of digested calories compared to the same exact food made at home. [Barr, Carmody] Processing the foods may break down food in a way that makes it easier for your body to digest and extract the energy from them.

Foods Digested Easily and Quickly (more likely to lead to weight gain)	Foods Digested Less Efficiently and Slowly (less likely to lead to weight gain)
Sugars Fats High glycemic carbs Processed foods	Protein (not processed) Low glycemic carbs Foods with a lot of fiber content

Calorie Balance

On any given day you fall into one of three categories:
- Calorie deficit (you digest less energy than you use)
  → lose body tissue
- Calorie balance
  (you digest about the same energy you use)
  → stay the same
- Calorie surplus (you digest more energy than you use)
  → gain body tissue

Most people who are reasonably active and eat naturally without paying too much attention will surprisingly not change their weight too much over time, meaning on average over many days they are in calorie balance. However, by paying more attention to your calorie intake and activity, you can try to create a calorie deficit or surplus with the following results:

Calorie deficit:
You will lose body tissue, which can be both fat and muscle. If you continue to stress your muscle frequently and maximally you will hopefully maintain most of your muscle mass and lose mainly fat. But you will still lose a small amount of muscle or create some damage without adequate repair.

Calorie surplus: You will gain body tissue, which can be both fat and muscle. If you continue to push yourself with your resistance workouts, you will hopefully gain some muscle. However, even though building muscle requires a fair amount of calories, the maximum amount of muscle that you can gain depends on your body's ability to repair and grow the muscle that you stress and damage during your workouts. As we mentioned in Chapter 3, growing muscle is a slow process that cannot really be sped up after a certain point. Once at its maximum, the speed of muscle growth cannot be increased by working out more or eating more. In other words, the average person may not be able to gain more than a pound of muscle a month no matter what they do. This also means that although you absolutely need to eat more calories to build those few pounds of muscle, any additional calories that you eat will be used to make fat. But how do you know the exact amount of calories you need to grow muscle without gaining fat? You do not. Therefore, you can err of the side of fewer calories, which means your muscle growth will be slower, or you can err on the side of more calories, which means your muscle growth will be as fast as allowed (still slow) and the extra calories will be used to make fat. That is why bodybuilders and actors, who are trying to gain as much muscle as possible very quickly, will accept that they will get fatter as well, and later go on a calorie deficit diet to "cut" the fat. It is also why some bodybuilders get frustrated and unfortunately start using steroids.

Let's look at an average sized person trying to gain muscle as fast as possible. Let's say this person can spend several hours a day working out. Let's say he genetically can gain 2lbs of muscle a month max. The muscle itself would take about 1800 x 2 = 3600 calories extra that month. It requires more when we take into account the inflammatory cells, the other cellular processes, and the repair of damaged muscle needed before new muscle can grow. So, let's estimate he actually needs an extra 5000-6000 calories a month to get an extra 2 pounds of muscle. That's about 160 to 200 extra calories every day. This does not seem like much, but you also need to add in the extra calories you need to do the workouts. Since he is working out several hours a day, trying to do as much micro muscle damage as possible, he may understandably need even an extra 200+ calories for each hour of the workout. (Harvard health) Of course the math becomes increasingly fuzzy and less precise as we try to estimate the total calories he should eat each day. Ultimately if he wants to get big as fast as possible, he will favor eating more rather than less, which means the extra calories may end up making fat. If he eats less than he needs, he may ultimately make less muscle that month.

This is why body builders alternate between bulking and cutting. In the bulking phase they err on the side of more. But the extra will go into fat. To minimize this, bulkers go on incredibly regimented high calorie diets of almost zero fat and only lean proteins (baked salmon, dry chicken breast, grains, quinoa, beans, etc.). If they eat less, they do not get their maximal muscle growth. Then, after several months of bulking they start to notice more body fat than they want, and they go into a cutting phase to lose the fat. During this time, they need to keep up the strength training to keep the muscles stimulated to stay strong. If not, the muscles will quickly get smaller. But even with working out at the same intensity, there will be some loss due to muscle damage and decreased ability to repair, so there is usually some loss in strength. Once again, they have to go on a very regimented diet. Most bodybuilders will tell you diet is 80% of the work. This is true if you need to look like a shredded body builder.

Unlike a bodybuilder or an actor, you are hopefully not trying to work out to look perfect on a specific day several months from now. You are trying to maintain the same healthy amount of muscle and a reasonably low amount of fat every day for the rest of your life. The way to achieve this is to consciously choose very mild amounts of calorie surplus when you want to gain muscle, and choose very mild amounts of calorie deficit when you want to lose fat. You have to choose one: gain muscle or lose fat and focus on doing this slowly with only a small calorie surplus or deficit. This allows you to gain muscle without gaining too much fat, and allows you to lose fat without losing too much muscle. Once you are in good shape, you simply need to maintain your routine and awareness to neither lose nor gain.

Can you gain muscle and lose fat simultaneously?
There are many trainers on the internet that will claim you can gain muscle and lose fat at the same time if you do everything right. There is no consistent method to do this and no proof that these regimens work. It is possible there is a physiological zone where this exists, but it is so narrow that it is impossible to find

on a daily basis. There are some studies that suggest it can occur over short periods of time (a few months at most) in beginners who just start resistance training. [Woods] There aren't any studies to suggest this can occur over longer periods of time or once a person has gained some extra muscle already.

In Summary: Food and your body

1. There are three types of food: carbohydrates, fats, and proteins. Proteins are the hardest to digest and the hardest to make.
2. The chemistry of your food can determine how many calories you actually absorb into your body, and how much your hunger is satisfied.
3. We frequently eat for reasons that have nothing to do with hunger or the need for energy.
4. When you eat more than your body needs, you gain fat. If you are stressing your muscle regularly, you can also repair and gain muscle. When you eat more, your aim is to maximize the muscle gain and minimize the fat gain.
5. When you eat less than your body requires, you can lose fat and muscle together. Your aim is to maximize the fat loss and minimize the muscle loss.
6. For practical purposes, in the long term you CANNOT gain muscle and lose fat at the same time.

Citations

1. Mattison JA, Colman RJ, Beasley TM, et al. Caloric restriction improves health and survival of rhesus monkeys. *Nat Commun.* 2017;8:14063. Published 2017 Jan 17. doi:10.1038/ncomms14063
2. Willcox BJ, Willcox DC, Todoriki H, et al. Caloric restriction, the traditional Okinawan diet, and healthy aging: the diet of the world's longest-lived people and its potential impact on morbidity and life span. *Ann N Y*

Acad Sci. 2007;1114:434-455. doi:10.1196/annals.1396.037

3. Pinker, Steven. Enlightenment Now: The case for reason, science, humanism, and progress, Chap 7: Sustenance. C.2018

4. Dunn R. The Hidden Truth about Calories. *Scientific American*, August 27, 2012.

5. Mattes RD, Kris-Etherton PM, Foster GD. Impact of peanuts and tree nuts on body weight and healthy weight loss in adults. *J Nutr.* 2008;138(9):1741S-1745S. doi:10.1093/jn/138.9.1741S

6. Barr SB, Wright JC. Postprandial energy expenditure in whole-food and processed-food meals: implications for daily energy expenditure. *Food Nutr Res.* 2010;54:10.3402/fnr.v54i0.5144. Published 2010 Jul 2. doi:10.3402/fnr.v54i0.5144

7. Carmody RN, Weintraub GS, Wrangham RW. Energetic consequences of thermal and nonthermal food processing. *Proc Natl Acad Sci U S A.* 2011;108(48):19199-19203. doi:10.1073/pnas.1112128108

8. http://www.health.harvard.edu/heart.Calories burned in 30 minutes for people of three different weights. Updated: August 13, 2018. Published: July, 2004

9. Wood PS, Krüger PE, Grant CC. DEXA-assessed regional body composition changes in young female military soldiers following 12-weeks of periodised training. *Ergonomics.* 2010;53(4):537-547. doi:10.1080/00140130903528160

Other References

1. Brownell KD, Horgan KB. Food Fight The Inside Story of the Food Industry, America's Obesity Crisis, and What We Can Do About. 2003

2. Corliss J. Break Through Your Set Point: How to Finally Lose the Weight You Want and Keep It Off. George Blackburn. 2008
3. Pollan M. In Defense of Food. 2008
4. Taubes G. Why We Get Fat: And What To Do About It. 2010

Chap 4. Using Resistance to build muscle

A Warning: Start Light

In the following chapter I am going to go over details of how to use resistance exercises to build muscle. If you are just starting, you have not used weights in a while, or you have an existing injury: Please start with very light weights for the first several workouts. Check your ego at the door, and DO NOT try to lift heavy weights right away. It is very easy to injure yourself. A simple tendinitis or disc bulge can set you back for months. Let your joints and tendons and stabilizing back and core muscles get used to the movements and mild resistance for the first several workouts before you start adding heavier weights.

The "science" of designing an ideal muscle building program

Unlike the science of understanding muscle and fat, there is no consistent science that determines the best schedule and regimen for working out. Most accepted routines are based on tradition, observations, and some empirical studies. Most studies involving weightlifting or exercise will involve taking two groups of participants (or the same group trying different ways), having them do everything identical except for one factor (the variable), and then making a conclusion about the variable based on the outcomes. For example, a typical study looking at how much rest is needed between sets will ask the participants to rest 1 minute, 3 minutes, and 5 minutes between sets and measure the weight they lift after rest. Based on this they will conclude that 1 minute is not enough, 3 minutes is enough to regain full strength, and 5 minutes is no better than 3. So, the recommendation will become "wait 3 min but not much more". However, when you look at the study, you will find the participants were 20-year-old intermediate or advanced lifters. So, does this apply to beginner to intermediate older lifters? Maybe beginners need to wait longer to get prepared mentally. Or maybe they need less because they are lifting less. Does it apply to people with minor injuries? Does it apply to 50 year old men?

Another problem with scientific studies is that when they use a small group of people, the studies are good at showing when a variable can make a big change in the outcome, but not good at proving when a variable can make a small change in the outcome. The study may claim they found "no difference" in the two groups, but in reality, if they ran the study on thousands of people rather than a dozen, they would find a difference. In addition, most studies are done over a few weeks or months, rather than years. This means there may be variables that help or hurt enough to make a difference over many years, but cannot always be shown in the way studies are designed. Or the benefit you see with the study at 4 weeks may disappear by 6 months.

Thus, most accepted regimens are not truly scientifically proven, but best guesses based on an assortment of random studies and personal long-term experience. Designing the program then ultimately depends on which variables are the most realistic, which outcomes are the most important, and how much time you are willing to devote to this. In our case, we are aiming to achieve a fit athletic build with as short a workout as possible.

Based on a variety of such studies, here are the variables and recommendations that need to be considered when designing a time efficient but effective workout using resistance training. I will review aerobic training in the next chapter.

1. Free weights vs machines.
2. Reps per set and amount of weight
3. Number of sets
4. Rest between sets
5. Frequency per week
6. Rest weeks

1. Free weights vs machines vs body weight vs bands

Free weights include barbells and dumbbells lifted against gravity. Machines usually involve movement restricted to hinges or tracks. This is one of the most studied topics around and when tested against each other, it is sometimes a tie, but almost always free weights come out ahead. The presumed advantages of free weights are that, in order to maintain stability, many more muscles are recruited during an individual exercise, including your core.

There may also be a bigger hormonal effect (i.e., more testosterone). There is better improvement in functional strength because it mimics everyday activities (squatting, lifting, etc.). There is proven improvement in sports performance. And finally, free weights usually burn more calories per movement.

The presumed advantages of machine weights are that they can target a specific muscle group more specifically, and they allow from some exercises that are nearly impossible with free weights (i.e., hip abduction and adduction, calf exercises).
They are safer if the weight is too heavy (you can't drop them) and do not require a spotter, making them less intimidating to a beginner. They are easier and quicker to adjust weights on.

Cable machines (which allow a bit more freedom than standard machines) probably fall somewhere between the two.

For this program I am going to strongly recommend free weights whenever possible.
Although intimidating to beginners, ultimately free weights will result in much more strength, muscle growth, and improved function for whatever time you put in. (Lopez, Bergquist) More muscles are recruited with each exercise. Almost every fitness expert will agree with this. In addition, when movements are restricted by tracks or hinges, they can lead to unnatural movements and injury. Most machine exercises require a lot more adjustment of seat and arm heights and levers to get the right movement. Machines can be very specific to a particular gym, while free weights are pretty much the same wherever you go. To overcome the initial fear of using barbells without a squatter, I am going to emphasize the need to build confidence by starting light, using a power cage, and paying attention to form. When you focus on good form rather than increasing the amount of weight, you will find free weights are not hard to use.

Covid 19 and Shelter in Place: Body weight, Resistance bands, and the Home Gym
Just as I was about to finish this book, I had to rethink my recommendations because of COVID 19 and shelter in place. Consequently, I had to take a closer look at the effectiveness of resistance exercises that we can do at home without having to purchase an entire home gym full of weights.

Body weight exercises include exercises such as pull ups, push-ups, dips, chin ups, squats, lunges, and other types of exercises that can be done with no weights. Band exercises involve movements that stretch and relax bands. The different colored bands can be combined to change the amount of resistance and tension. The literature suggests that these exercises can be just as effective as weights in increasing strength and muscle mass. Some band companies will try to claim that because resistance bands offer their greatest resistance when your muscles are at maximal contraction, they are more effective than weights at increasing muscle. Although it is true that resistance bands do increase resistance progressively as you contract, there is no evidence to suggest this is superior. However, in multiple short-term studies, both body weight exercises and resistance bands are as effective at building muscle as free weights for beginners.

The major advantage of body weight and band exercises is that you do not have to go to the gym, and you can figure out a way to do them almost anywhere. Another advantage is that they are less intimidating than using free weights for the first time, and you are perhaps less likely to injure yourself compared to using free weights.

What are the disadvantages of using body weight exercises and resistance band exercises? **The huge disadvantage of these exercises is that it is very difficult to fine tune the weight, which makes it much harder to design a time efficient work out, and makes it much harder to make small amounts of progress between workouts.** The other problem with resistance bands is that the exact resistance is difficult to reproduce from one day to another because small changes in the setup or length of the bands can change the actual resistance by a lot.

As an example, let's look at trying to improve leg strength by doing squats. If you squat using a barbell (or even by holding dumbbells on each side) you should pick a weight that will stress your muscles maximally in the 8 to 12 rep range. I will explain why I choose this range in the next section.   In the beginning you may be only able to do 8 to 9 reps, but after a few weeks or months you may be able to do 12 reps consistently. Based on this, you can clearly see that you have improved your strength and made progress, and you can think about adding another 5, 10, or maybe 20 lbs. Even small increases in your reps or your total weight confirm that you are making consistent progress and that your routine is working and consistently pushing you to your limit. Similarly, if you are trying to lose weight, you may lose some strength, but you will know by how much. Now, let's try to get the same results with squats using body weight only, or resistance bands. If you use your body weight only, you may find that you can do perhaps 10, 20 or 30 or eventually even 40 squats before you give up. This may be effective, but it is not time efficient. If you use resistance bands, you might have trouble finding the right combination of bands to get you in the 8 to 12 rep range. You might find yourself doing more than 12 with a certain combination of bands, but dropping down to 4 to 6 reps when you add one more band to increase the resistance. If the width of your feet standing on the bands changes a bit from one day to the next, you will not be working with the same resistance consistently.

Similarly, if you are doing pull ups to improve your back, some of you might find that you can do much less than 8. Even if you do only a few in the beginning, you will still improve over time, but you will not be getting the most out of each workout. Therefore, your progress might be slower compared to using free weights in the right rep range.

Therefore, if you want to gain strength and muscle mass in the most time efficient routine possible, I am going to strongly recommend free weights whenever possible. This means using dumbbells at minimum, and ideally both dumbbells and barbells.

If social distancing or other reasons make going to a gym impossible, then I would recommend trying to get some weights for home use. Barbells, Power cages, and Bench press sets are expensive and require lots of space and are unrealistic for most of us. However, you should be able to make reasonable progress with at least some adjustable dumbbells and a relatively inexpensive reclining bench. During the pandemic I found I was still able to do most of my exercises and make progress with adjustable dumbbells ($200), an adjustable bench ($150), a doorway pull-up bar, and a dip station (for both inverse rows and dips). Although I did not push myself as hard as with barbells and a power cage at the gym, I was able to make similar progress by adding some extra exercises and time to my dumbbell workouts. After all, working out at home usually gives you a little bit of extra time by not having to travel to the gym.

2.   Reps (repetitions) per set, amount of weight, and form.

Reps are the number of times you can lift a weight before having to quit. Your **one rep max** is the highest weight you can lift at least once. Obviously, you will be able to complete more reps with a low weight and less reps with a higher weight. There is no clear-cut study that suggests one way is better than the other. Some stress the idea that weight must be at least 70% of your one rep max to have an effect. Others stress the need to keep the muscle under tension for at least 30-40 secs (with a two second contraction and two second relaxation this usually means 10-12 reps). Others stress that pushing the muscle to anaerobic fatigue (the burn) is what matters. **The movement should be slow and controlled throughout, and not depend on momentum or bounce. There should be no jerky**

movements. This makes sure the muscles you are trying to isolate are doing all the work.

In general, it is accepted (though not clearly proven) that lifting very heavy weights in a low rep range (1-6) will primarily improve strength (strength training), heavy weights in a mid rep range (8-12) will increase muscle size (muscle building), and light weights in the high rep range (over 12) will improve endurance. However, there is a fair amount of overlap between strength training and muscle building training: both will increase strength and muscle size to some degree.

Finally, there is a clear benefit to lifting through the full range of motion: allowing the muscle to go from as much extension (stretched) to as much flexion (squeezed) as possible. Most trainers suggest trying to consciously contract and "squeeze" the muscle at the end of flexion. This is the most time efficient way of giving your muscle the maximal workout. Work is defined as weight x distance moved, so the most efficient use of time is to maximize the distance you move the weight. You want as many actin myosin interactions as possible. You may see some people lifting through a very limited range of motion. Either they are doing it wrong because they are eager to add more weight, or they are doing "finishing" exercises to target a very specific part of their muscle. This is only a move for bodybuilders trying to get a very specific shape to their muscle, gym rats with loads of extra time, or beginners who don't understand the importance of full range.

For this program I recommend a rep range of 8-12 with a full range of motion for the following reasons
- Using very heavy free weights in the lower rep range can be intimidating
- It is much more difficult to maintain good form and a full

range of motion with heavier weights. The tendency is to sacrifice form when lifting too heavy.

- Using very heavy free weights in the lower rep range has a higher risk of injury in older men, especially on the low back.
- Using very heavy weights requires much more mental focus with every workout, which tends to lead to more inconsistencies between workouts and difficulty measuring progress.

3.   Number of sets

Most programs will suggest somewhere between 3 to 5 sets of an exercise, and like many aspects of weight training, much of this is based on tradition as much as science. When studied it seems that 3 sets consistently promote more muscle growth than 1, and 5 sets promotes even more, but not by that much. In addition, you may be able to gain increased strength (with less growth) with an even shorter workout. (Scholenfield) So the question becomes: is doing 5 sets instead of 3 really worth the extra time? If you have the time, it probably is. If you do not, it probably isn't. The good news is that for most men, doing 10 sets may actually be worse due to overtraining and excess muscle damage. Thank goodness.

For this program I am going to recommend one very light set (12 reps), one medium set (12 reps), and three max sets (8 - 12 reps). If you really have the time you could increase your max sets to 4 or 5, but you are probably better off using the time to do some of the optional exercises or an aerobic session.

The purpose of the first very light set (light enough to do 20 reps if you wanted to) is to focus entirely on range of motion and perfect form. This is followed by a medium weight set (50-80%

of your eventual max) to focus on form and prepare yourself for the heavier weight. After this you should pick a weight that will challenge you in the 8-12 range (we will call this your max set). With each max set you should feel like you are really giving everything you have to do the last one or two reps, while still maintaining good form and full range. If you can do more than twelve reps in any one set, you need to increase the weight. If you can't do 8 on any one set, you need to decrease the weight. If you can do 12 on your first set but less than 8 on your last, you need to rest more between sets.

4.   Rest between sets

Here the studies are pretty consistent. If you are pushing yourself with higher weights, the more rest the better. (Senna) After 3 to 5 minutes on average, most studies do not show much more benefit to waiting longer. Of course, there is individual variation. When you first start, I would recommend waiting at least 3 minutes, and even longer if you feel much weaker with each set. Personally, I find that when you first start it's a good idea to pay attention to how long you are resting, but over time you get a good sense of when you are ready to go again without wasting too much time waiting. In addition to being physically rested, it's important to feel mentally ready for the next set. If you go into the next set confident that you'll finish your set, you almost always will. If you go into it doubting yourself that doubt only grows with each rep and you may tend to quit earlier.

5.   Frequency per week

After a workout, muscle repair and recovery start right away and will continue for several days. Many routines are based on maximally working out one muscle group (i.e., just back or just chest or just legs) and then waiting an entire week before working them out again. If you truly push that muscle group to the maximum that day, it may truly take a week for that muscle group to repair, grow, and recover, and still gain. However, most of us cannot consistently push our muscles to the maximum amount of microtrauma with each workout to justify a full week of rest, and we end up gaining at a much slower rate than working each group more often. The once a week schedule also locks you into having to work out that muscle group on the same day every week. The vast majority of muscle repair and recovery occurs in the first 48 hours, after which they can be stressed maximally once more. Growth actually occurs well beyond that, but exercising the muscles again after 48 or 72 hours does not impair growth. Working on each muscle group more frequently allows for more consistent progress and growth, even if you have days when you do not put in your maximum 100 percent effort. It also allows for a much more flexible schedule. And most importantly, the studies back it up: twice a week training almost always leads to faster growth and strength gains than once a week.

It is also generally accepted (but not proven) that bicep and triceps workouts need to be added only once a week since they are being worked during the back and chest exercises already.

6.   Rest weeks

It is unclear if taking a complete week off from lifting any weights really helps, but having such a rest week once every 6 to 8 weeks does not seem to hurt. Most studies suggest that one week of rest does not decrease strength. This is assuming you still remain otherwise active and maintain a healthy diet during that week. For some people, a week's rest allows you to come back fresher and stronger. For others, breaking the routine for even a week makes it harder to come back mentally. If you often find it difficult to resume a program when you stop for a short time, I personally recommend forcing yourself to have a rest week and learning how to convince yourself to resume your routine when the rest week is over. Learning how to do this will make it easier in the future to restart your routine if life forces you to stop it for a while.

Because there is no clear science on the rest week, I recommend taking a rest week intermittently during those times that following your routine is more challenging than usual. I will save my rest week for an extremely busy week, or during a week when I am on vacation or travelling. As long as your rest week occurs less than once every two months, you will be fine and not lose any of the progress you made.

The Exercise Program: The Schedule

Here is a typical schedule over a 7 to 9 day cycle. Essentially it is a weekly schedule, but I allow for a possible 9-day interval to provide additional flexibility. Each cycle involves the following:

Resistance Workout 1: Heavy Weight (Barbell or dumbbell)

This is the base workout using the heaviest weights which leads to the most progress. If you can only do one workout a week, this is it. Once you get in decent shape, doing this workout only even once a week will maintain your strength. In general, a barbell will allow you to use the most weight and push you the most. If you do not have access to barbell weights, then you can use dumbbells instead.

Body part	Exercise
legs	Barbell Squat or Dumbbell squat
back	Deadlift (with barbell or dumbbells) or Dumbbell row
chest	Bench press (incline or flat) or dumbbell chest press.
shoulders	Shoulder press (barbell or dumbbell)

Resistance Workout 2

Like the 1st workout, this workout will also involve your legs, your back, your chest, and your shoulders. However, it involves lighter weights like dumbbells, body weights, bands, or even machines if that is what you prefer. There are a lot of options for exercises in this workout, and you can choose the exercises that you prefer, as long as you choose at least one exercise for each body part.

Body part	Exercise examples
legs	Lunge, single leg squats
back	Barbell row, dumbbell row, pull ups, inverted rows
chest	Incline or flat dumbbell press, diamond dumbbell press, pushups, dips
shoulders	Dumbbell shoulder press, Lateral dumbbell raises

Resistance (+) X-tra Add-On Workout: OPTIONAL A La Carte Exercises

On any days you have extra time, these exercises can be added on to Workout 1 or 2 the same day. Or they can be done the very next day after Workout 1 or Workout 2. If you want to continue to work the larger muscle groups you can do body weight exercises like pull ups, push-ups, and dips. Or you can work on your arms and calves. These exercises will give your muscles a little extra wear and tear to improve your growth, but they do not require the high weight and full strength and effort of the main workouts. For the extra add on workout, work on whatever you feel like and based on whatever time permits. Once again, think of these exercises as a bit of an extra boost to your progress, but not mandatory.

Body part	Exercise examples
Full body	Barbell power clean, farmer's walk
legs	Calf machine, adductor/abductor machines
back	Pull ups, inverted rows
chest	Push-ups, dips, dumbbell flye
shoulders	Shoulder dumbbell flye
triceps	Skull crushers, triceps press
biceps	Incline curls, barbell curls, dumbbell curls
Abdomen, core	Crunches, captain's chair, planks, etc.

Resistance Workout Schedule
Wait a minimum of 36 hours between the end of the first resistance workout (+X-tra if added) and beginning of the 2nd resistance workout. And then another minimum of 36 hours between the 2nd workout (+X-tra if added) and your next cycle, starting with the 1st workout. On average you will be doing the two workouts each week, spaced apart as much as possible.

Preferably you want 48 hours or more of rest between the weight workouts, but you can compress it to 36 hours depending on your schedule. In the beginning, I would recommend resting as long as possible if your muscles feel very sore, since this means they may need more time for repair.

Here are some random examples of what your schedule could look like. The schedule can differ from week to week as long as you get enough rest between the heavy weight workouts and do not go into workout 1 or 2 feeling sore. You can see that you have a lot of options as long as you are willing to find time for at least two weight workouts during the week.

WEEK	Day 1	Day 2	Day 3	Day 4	Day 5	Day 6	Day 7
Example 1	1	rest	rest	2	rest	rest	rest
Example 2	1	rest	rest	2	X	rest	rest
Example 3	1	rest	2	rest	X	rest	rest
Example 4	1	rest	X	rest	2	rest	rest
Example 5	1	X	rest	2	X	rest	rest
Example 6	1 + X	rest	rest	2 + X	rest	rest	rest

Compared to many other programs the schedule may seem

confusing, but unlike other programs that are built around a very fixed schedule every 7 days, this program allows you the flexibility of adjusting your schedule while still maximizing muscle growth between sessions.

In this program you try to work each big muscle group at least twice a week (or 9 days) without stressing each group to the maximum and risking injury, but still promoting muscle repair and strengthening before the next session.

Here are some examples: If you can only make it to the gym twice that week, if your Workout 1 is on Saturday, your Workout 2 can be on Monday, Tuesday, or Wednesday. If the next week you can make it to the gym 4 days that week, you can do your Workout 1 Sunday, an X tra workout Monday, the Workout 2 on Wed, and another X tra workout on Thursday. A beginner can usually make good progress with the minimum schedule alone. Eventually, putting more time in will lead to better progress. On the weeks you have the time for more frequent sessions, you can really boost your progress. The advantage of this program over others is you can have a fair amount of variation from week to week and still make progress, or at least maintain the progress you have made.

As mentioned before, you do not have to plan rest weeks, but if you have a week where it is difficult to make it to the gym, consider it a rest week. Try to keep them fewer than once every 6 to 8 weeks. During your rest week, even if you cannot get to weights, try to do some aerobic activity if possible and pay particular attention to your diet so you do not gain fat.

Resistance Workout Reps and Sets
Every weight exercise is going to be done with a low weight and medium weight warm up, followed by 3 sets of high weights.

Set Low x 1:   12 - 15 reps of light warm up

Use just the bar or a very light weight to focus entirely on form. You could do 20 if you had to. Make a conscious effort to maintain the very same form for all the remaining sets getting as much extension and contraction as possible.

Set Med x 1:   12 reps of a medium weight: about 50-80% of your high weight.

This set allows you to reinforce your form and gets you physically and mentally prepared for the full effort you will need for the higher weight. The 12th rep should feel like a bit of a struggle. You could do perhaps 13 or 14 if you had to, but not much more.

Set High x 3:   8-12 reps per set of your high weight, for three sets.

When you first start, pick a weight that you think you could do about 10 max and do as many reps as possible until you cannot complete another rep with complete form.

If you can do more than 12 on any one set, you need to increase the weight.

If you cannot do 8 on any one set, you need to decrease the weight.

The last one or two reps of each set should be a struggle, and you should end each set convinced you could not possibly do one more. Fatigue, soreness, and failure in the muscle you are working on should be your rate limiting factor.

If you are dropping off a lot between sets (i.e., 12 on the first set but less than 8 on the last), try to rest more between sets.

Keep track of your weight and how many reps you do with each set, so you can monitor progress and plateaus. When you can consistently complete at least 10 reps on the last set, think about increasing the weight for next time by just a little.

Aerobic/Cardio 1 & 2 (&3 if possible)

Two to three separate sessions of 10-30 min, your choice. Can be HIIT (high intensity interval training) or at a steady pace. See the next chapter to understand the hype about HIIT. If you do a 10 min session, it should be a HIIT session. If you do a 20 to 30 minute session, it can be either HIIT or at a steady pace.

Examples of aerobic activity include running, elliptical, stationary bike, swimming, rowing machine, stair climber, jump rope, etc.

The aerobic exercise session can be done on any day (a weight day or a rest day), as long as you complete at least two sessions over the 7 to 9 days. If you can add a third session during the 7-9 days, your cardiovascular endurance will improve faster.

The Exercise Program: Keeping Track of Progress

Keeping track of your progress is the single most important part of any routine you adopt. If you do not keep track, you have no way of knowing if you are doing your workouts correctly and when you might need to make an adjustment. When you first start, hopefully you will increase your strength quickly, but eventually you will hit a natural plateau for your size and age, after which progress is much slower but every little bit still matters. Sometimes when you are more focused on fat loss, you may see some loss of strength.

I recommend sticking with the same exercises every time you do the workout for several months so you can measure progress over time. Definitely try to keep a good record of the heavy weight barbell or dumbbell exercises you do in Workout 1. If your Workout 2 also involves dumbbell exercises, keep close track of those as well.

Whenever you have some extra time at the end of a workout add in some additional exercises, focusing on any part of your body that is the weakest. When you add in some additional exercises, feel free to mix them up and try different ones. You do not need to worry too much about progress with these last additional exercises since you will be doing them intermittently and inconsistently at the end of your overall workout, and your strength may vary every time you do them.

I keep track of my progress on an excel file on my smartphone. If you are old school, you can just use a paper printout and pen instead.

I divide my excel file into two tabs: schedule and weights. (you can download an excel file at www.facebook.com/getstronglifelong)

SCHEDULE: Sample Worksheet.
- This page keeps track of which exercises I did on each day.
- The rows are days in the month, and the columns are the individual exercises.
- This example shows a primarily barbell and dumbbell workout over two weeks. You can put the exercises you do most commonly in the columns.

	BARBELL WORKOUT				DUMBELL WORKOUT				XTRA WTS			XTRA BODY			XTRA CORE			AEROBIC	COMMENTS
	squat	dd lift	bench	press	lunge	row	chest	shoulder	hip thrust	tricep	biceps	calf	pullups	pushups	dips	crunch	bicycle		
1. Sa	x	x	x	x															
Sun																			
Mon																		run 2 miles	
Tues					x	x	x	x											
Wed									x	x		x							
Thur																		st bike 30 min	
Fri																			
2. Sa																			
Sun	x	x	x	x															
mon																		run 2 miles	
Tues																			
Wed					x	x	x	x	x										
Thur																			
Fri																		st bike 30 min	
3. Sa	x	x	x	x															
Sun							x	x	x										
Mon																		st bike 30 min	
Tues																			
Wed					x	x	x	x				x							
Thurs													x	x				st bike 30 min	
Fri																			
4. Sat	x	x	x	x															

WEIGHT: Sample worksheet

- This page keeps track of my reps and weights for each exercise.
- Each column is a month and rows have all the exercises I want to see progress in. I do not put in exercises I do rarely or inconsistently.
- With each workout I update the latest weights and reps for that exercise under the current month.
- When using a barbell (which is 45lbs), you can just enter the weight you add to the barbell, or if you prefer, you can add 45lbs and record the total weight.
- When the month is over, I start entering into the next month's column.
- Columns from the prior months will show me the amount of weight I lifted previously at the end of that month. Hopefully I can see some progress over several months.
- It is sometimes helpful to add a row for your own body weight if you want to see progress gaining muscle or

losing fat.

- This sample shows the progress over 4 months for barbell exercises.

	Sept	Oct	Nov	Dec	Jan	
weight (lbs)	170	171	172	171		
Squat-barbel	80 x 12	80x12	80 x 12	80 x12		
	100 x 10,9,8	100 x10,10,8	100 x12,11,10	120 x9,8,8		
Dead lift	70 x12	70 x12	70 x12	90 x12		
	110 x12,10,10	120x 10,8,8	120 x 11,10,10	140 x 9,9,8		
inc bench	50 x12	50 x12	60 x12	60 x12		
	70 x9,9,8	70 x11,10,10	80 x10,10,8	80 x11,10,10		
shldr press	30x12	30 x12	30 x12	40 x12		
	50 x8,8,8	50x10,8,8	50 x10,10,10	70 x9,8,8		
lunge	30x12	30 x12	40 x12	50 x12		
	40 x 10,8,8	40 x 12,12,11	60 x 10,9,8	60 x 12,11,11		

The Essential Barbell Exercises: Squat, Deadlift, Bench Press, Overhead Press.

Barbell Exercises and the Power Cage

- The standard Olympic barbell found in most gyms weighs about 45lbs just by itself. So, don't feel bad if you are not adding too much weight to it when you first start.
- For the barbell exercises it is going to be very hard to have confidence and make progress without the safety of a power cage or a spotter in case you fail. A power cage is a large rectangular cage that allows you to place the bar on hooks at the right starting height, and adjustable bars on the side that will catch the bar at your lowest point if you can no longer lift it. You should use a power cage for the squat and probably even the bench press in

the beginning until you have the confidence to no longer need it. It will give you the confidence to push yourself further, knowing you will not kill yourself if you fail.

Legs: Barbell Squat

- You place a weighted barbell on your upper back, go from standing to squatting, and then back up to standing. Try to squat at least until your thighs are parallel to the ground, or lower as long as your knees don't hurt. This is much more important than the amount of weight you use. As you increase the weight you will not want to squat as low, so try to still focus on form and lighten the weight if you find yourself shortening your movement. Make sure to contract your gluteal muscles at the end of each lift when you are standing.
- Set your feet apart about shoulder width, but use your light weights or no weights to determine the most comfortable positions for your feet. Widening your stance will work your inner thigh muscles more.
- Set up the power cage so you can place the bar safely on your back without having to tiptoe. Set the lower side bars to catch the barbell at the lowest portion of your squat, using an unloaded barbell bar to guide you.
- Place the bar on your upper back on the top part of your shoulder blades and not your lower neck. Keep your grip (palms facing forward) as narrow as possible. The narrow grip forces your back muscles (the upper trapezius and rhomboids) to squeeze and support the bar instead of your bones.
- Try to prevent your knees from moving too forward or your back from flexing down Look upward to keep your neck slightly extended, which prevents you from flexing. If you look at your profile in a mirror, the bar should be

going almost straight up and down and not forward or back. The bar should be moving in a line directly above your feet, not in front of it. In the beginning you can actually put a bench or chair behind you and sit down on it, since the movement should almost be like sitting down and getting up.

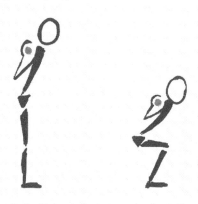

Back and Legs: Deadlift

- You place a weighted barbell on the floor in front of you and lift it off the floor until you are standing, back extended a bit, and then place it back down again. The bar usually starts a few inches off the floor because of the weights placed on the sides. You can bend your knees just enough to grab the bar and keep your low back straight (not curled) as you lift. You can lower the bar again all the way to the floor, or just an inch or two off the floor before lifting again.) Grab the bar with a shoulder width grip or slightly wider.
- If you feel a bit of a jolt every time you lower the weight back to the ground, place two soft yoga mats under each of the weights. This will give you some shock absorption but try not to bounce it back.
- The normal grip with palms facing in (pronated) should be enough for the lighter weights, but for most people is

a rate limiting factor for the higher weights.

- If the grip is limiting you, switch to either a hook grip (your front fingers go over your thumb, and your thumb will hurt) or an alternating grip with one palm facing in and one palm facing out (one pronated, one supinated). Make sure to keep the palm out arm slightly tense to prevent tearing the biceps, and alternate which palm faces out between sets.
- Make sure to extend your back and contract your gluteals at the end of each lift when you are standing.

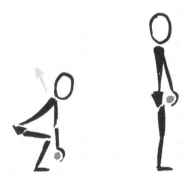

Chest: Bench Press (usually incline)

- You lie facing up on a bench, grab a weighted bar off the rack with hands a bit wider than your shoulders, bring the bar down to your chest (or as close as possible) and then lift straight up towards the ceiling. A very wide grip will reduce your strength, but a narrow grip may hurt your shoulders. Adjust the width of your grip until you can lower the bar as close to your chest as possible without your shoulder joints bothering you.
- The incline (angled) bench press works out the upper and inner chest more than the flat bench press. Although most people can lift more with a flat bench press, this is the one exercise where I might recommend going with

the exercise that gives you a better proportional look rather than better strength. Especially for those of us who struggle with man boobs.

- Most incline benches are fixed at around 30 degrees. If adjustable, the bench should be adjusted between 15 to 45 degrees. The more upright the angle, the more the workout involves the upper chest and shoulders, but the less weight that can be lifted. Adjust the incline to feel the workout in your upper chest.
- There is never a reason to do a decline bench press.
- Experiment with the width of your grip frequently to see what allows you to lift the most.
- Try to have the bar touch your chest or come as close as possible to guarantee a full range of movement.

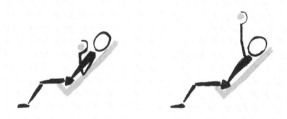

Shoulders: Barbell lift

- You lift a weighted barbell (long or short) off the floor and over your head. Your grip width should be slightly wider than your chest. Bring the bar down in front of you as close as possible to your upper chest (below your chin), then lift up again and make sure to contract your deltoids.

Other Leg, Back, Chest, and Shoulder Exercise Examples

Most of the exercises below are well known by name alone, so my descriptions about the actual exercises themselves will be kept as short as possible. If you are still confused about the movement, I would recommend looking them up on the internet or another source. Always pay attention to maintaining proper form to avoid injury.

Leg Exercises
- Barbell front squat

    o You hold the barbell on your upper chest with your palms facing out. (I personally do not like this exercise because the stress on the wrists is much harder on older men.)
- Straight leg deadlift.
    o This is a deadlift with legs completely straight and lowering the bar as far down as possible without arching your back. This will target the hamstrings and gluteal muscles, but can be hard on anyone with low back problems. In fact, you must keep the back arches and not let it flex for the exercise to be effective. It is better to use a lighter weight or not do the exercise at all if this is a problem.
- Alternating lunges.
    o Lunges will target the anterior legs muscles (quads) more than the posterior ones.
    o Use a short barbell placed on your back (like the barbell squat) or hold dumbbells to your side.
    o Lunges can be done moving forward or in place.

    o Bring the back leg knee close to the ground or touch the ground briefly.
    o The front leg is the one doing the lifting. Extend the leg and contract the glutes fully at the top of the lift.
- Bench single leg lunges

- Place your back foot on a bench or chair and perform all your reps with the front leg. Then switch. This usually requires more balance than regular lunges.
- Step ups.
  - Step ups, like lunges, will target the anterior quadriceps muscles the most
  - There are many variations of the exercise, but all involve stepping up on a bench or chair. Start with a low height and no weight. Eventually try to get to a height where your hip is at least 90 degrees at the start
  - The most important element is to come up and down slowly and not drop onto the floor. Use the front leg to do all the work
- Dumbbell squat
  - Take the dumbbell you will be lifting and place it on the floor vertically. Place two more dumbbells vertically (or two short step stools) on each side, and stand on these dumbbells/step stools while you squat and, holding the dumbbell by the end and not the middle, lift the middle dumbbell straight up until standing straight.
- Jump lunges.

Gluteal Exercises
- Hip thrust (raise) with barbell.
  - This is probably the single best exercise to specifically stress the large gluteal muscles and your hamstrings. This is a tricky exercise to set up, and I recommend looking up internet videos to get the proper form. You need to sit upright on the floor with your back against a bench. The edge of the bench should be on the lowest portion of

your scapula. Put your legs out straight and take a barbell with weights and roll it over your legs until the center of the bar is in the middle of your pelvis (the midportion of the bar should be somewhere between your belly button and your pubic bone). You need a very thick padding between your pelvis and the bar. You have to use padding, or the bar is just too painful. Now thrust your hips up into the air until your knees are at 90 degrees and the rest of your body is relatively flat and in line. Make sure to look forward. If you look up or away, you can arch your back which will not help your glutes and only hurt your back. If you look forward always towards your knees you will automatically isolate the gluteal muscles. Hold the bar at the top for a few seconds, then sit back down and repeat.

Back Exercises
- Barbell bent over row
  - Bend over almost 45 to 90 degrees, legs straight, avoid flexing the back, and bring a weighted barbell up to the chest and then back down. Proper form is critical, so I recommend looking on the internet for examples of good form.
- Single dumbbell row
  - Bracing your right hand and right knee on a flat bench, use your left arm to lift a dumbbell from a straight hanging arm to a row, with the dumbbell up to the side of the chest, and then back down again. Then switch sides.
- Wide grip pull-up
  - Pull up with palms out and a slightly wider than shoulder grip.

- This is one of the best exercises for the latissimus dorsi
- If you need help, use the help of a weighted pull up machine.
- If you can do more than 12 with each set, you may need to add weight using a weight belt.

Chest Exercises
- Incline dumbbell press
  - The tricky part is getting the dumbbells into position. Once again you can use a flat bench or an incline bench at 15 to 45 degrees. Sit forward on the bench and hold the dumbbells resting on your knees. As you lie back onto the bench, keep your hips and knees bent and use your knees to lift the dumbbells into place by the side of your chest (one knee at a time for heavy weights), lower your legs back into the usual position, and then lift the weights just like a bench press. Once done, bring your knees back up to stabilize the dumbbells as you sit forward and then let them down.

- Squeeze incline dumbbell press
  - This press will specifically target the inner upper

pecs, which is often hard to develop. In complete honesty, this is a vanity exercise since there is no real health reason to make the inner pecs stronger. For this press, make sure the two dumbbells should be parallel to each other with both ends touching. Your palms are facing inward as you hold them, squeezing the dumbbells together, like the end of a fly movement. Keep the dumbbells touching at all times as you lower them to your chest and then raise them to the top. Another variation involves putting a soft foam or medicine ball between the dumbbells, forcing you to squeeze the ball to keep it in place.

- Push ups
  - You can vary the width of your arms to change the exercise. Putting your hands closer together targets the triceps and inner chest more. If you cannot do enough, start with modified push-ups with your knees on the ground at all times. If you can do more than 12 with each set, you may need to add some weight to your back.

- Dips
  - Dips are great for the chest and especially the triceps. Try to maintain full range by dipping down as low as possible and make sure to squeeze your triceps at the top. Once again you can use a weighted dip assist machine if you need help to do enough. If you can do more than 12 with each set, you may need to add weight using a weight belt.

Shoulder
- Dumbbell lift
  - Bring the dumbbells down to your shoulders, and raise the dumbbells above your head with arms

fully extended. Try to contract your deltoids at the end of the movement. Your elbows can be out to your side or in front of you. Putting the elbows in front of you will work your anterior deltoids more than your posterior ones.

- Dumbbell flye
  - Place the dumbbells by the side of your body near your hips with palms facing in, and keeping your arms straight, lift your arm out like you are "Flying". Your palms will be holding the weights facing the floor. Hold them for a second or two at the top of the movement before lowering them slowly again.

Full body exercises
- Burpees
- Kettlebell swings
- Farmers carry
  - Pick up heavy dumbbells in each hand and try to walk as far as possible with medium sized steps for at least 40 secs per set. Count your steps, and try to increase your weight or the number of steps as you progress.
- Clean and Press
  - Start with a short barbell on the floor, pull it up to your chest. At this point you will have to shift from a palm down to a palm up grip, and push the barbell above your head. The exercise is like a combination of a deadlift and a barbell lift. Some variations add a squat just after the change in grip. The hardest part of this exercise is usually the change in grip and the stress it might put on the wrist for those with weak grips or any type of carpal tunnel symptoms. If you find the exercise

is hard on your wrists, use lighter weights with more reps rather than risk injury.

Calf and Arm Exercise Examples

Working the big muscles (legs, back, chest) twice a week will automatically give your smaller muscles (calves, arms) a sufficient workout. If you feel you want more growth on your calves and arms, or you find that your smaller muscles are limiting your big muscle exercises, then add calf and arms to your workout once a week. Doing them more than once a week may actually backfire by causing fatigue and limiting your big muscle workout, which is much more important to overall muscle growth and strength.

As I mentioned before, working the muscle through the maximum range of motion will lead to the best results. For smaller muscles this often means starting the exercise with the muscle as stretched as possible.

Calves

Unlike all the other exercises, calf exercises are hard to do without a machine. The calf consists of the more obvious gastrocnemius muscles which are the two rounded muscles on each side, and the soleus muscle which is a deeper longer muscle down the middle.

- Straight leg calf raises
  - These will work both gastrocnemius and soleus.
  - Most gyms have some type of calf machine where you stand straight, the weight is applied to your shoulders, and you place the balls of your feet at the edge of a platform.
- Donkey calf raises
  - These involve flexing at the hip 90 degrees or more and applying weight to your low back /bottom.

- These place the gastrocnemius on more stretch and give them a better workout than the straight leg
- Seated calf raises
  - This exercise involves sitting with knees flexed 90 degrees and applying the weight to the top of the knees
  - Because the gastrocnemius muscles are attached to the front of the knee, bending the knee completely relaxes them. This exercise only works the soleus, and therefore is probably not worth the time compared to the straight or donkey raise.

Triceps

The triceps muscle is actually more responsible for bigger arms than the bicep and is equally important to overall strength and function. So, if you are short on time, choose triceps over biceps

- Skull crushers with stretch.
  - Using a short barbell, lie down on a bench with your head at the very end of the bench. Lift the barbell above your chest with a relatively close grip, and keeping your elbows straight, pivot towards your head until your triceps are fully stretched. This is your starting point. Now let your elbows bend and lower the weight down towards the top of or behind your head. Try not to actually hit your head (hence the name). Now go back to the starting point by contracting your triceps. Squeeze at the end but keep them stretched.
- Dips with a shoulder width grip (elbows close to body)
- Narrow grip bench press
  - Keep your hands as close together as possible towards the center of the barbell bar. Use a short barbell if a long one is hard to balance.

Biceps
- Incline dumbbell curls.
  - Sit on an incline bench with a 45-degree angle and let the arms drop down to the floor for the beginning of the movement. This will stretch the long head of the biceps, giving you the maximum range of motion with each curl.
  - Rotate your wrist to what is most comfortable. If the palm up grip leads to pain at the elbow or tendonitis, it may be easier to switch to a hammer grip (thumb side facing up).
- Standing or seated dumbbell curls
- Barbell curls
- Chin ups. These are Pull ups with palms facing towards you and arms shoulder width apart

Core and Abdominal Exercises

The obsession with "six pack abs" has flooded the internet with all sorts of routines and exercises promising to get you some. Moderate muscle definition helps, but ultimately you need to have low total body fat to have them show through. If you already have very little body fat, AND you would like some more bulk to your abdominal muscles, AND you have the extra time, then it is probably worthwhile adding some core (abdominal) specific exercises to your weekly routine.

Otherwise, I would say abdominal exercises should probably be the lowest priority exercise you do for the following reasons:
- When done incorrectly, they can lead to lower back injury.
- The squats and deadlifts will strengthen your core by themselves
- Many types of aerobic exercises (like rowing or biking)

can also strengthen your core

- Core exercises will not reduce the fat inside your abdomen or around your belly. They may improve the tone of your abdominal muscles and your overall posture, but they will not decrease your waist size.
- You are better off focusing your time and energy on the other workouts to burn overall fat in your body.

If you do have the extra time and/or enjoy doing them (very few people do), there are two forms of core specific exercises: planks and crunches.

The basic plank involves facing the ground supported on either completely straight arms, or on your elbows (hands together in front of you) while you try to keep your spine and legs in a completely straight line, usually for 30 seconds to 2 minutes*. Because the muscle is not contracting and stretching through its full range of motion, the basic plank probably will not lead to much abdominal muscle growth. It can, however, improve your overall posture and total body strength.

The basic midline crunch involves lying on your back and pressing your ribs towards your belly button, raising your chest above the ground slightly, keeping your back and neck straight, and then lowering slowly still using the abdominal muscles. This crunch works your rectus abdominus muscles, which is the central muscle that leads to that six pack look. The crunch should theoretically build your rectus more than the plank, because you are at least putting the muscle through some range of motion. However, in reality it is not a very practical exercise.

Bicycle crunches involve crossing your right elbow to your left knee, and vice versa, to work your lateral abdominal muscles (obliques and transverse) and your central muscles. It is a more practical movement than the midline crunch, because it helps develop the core strength you need for rotational movement in activities like swimming, wood chopping, throwing, batting, swinging a racquet, and bicycling.

Finally, we come back to the plank. Although the basic plank does not involve any range of motion, there are many variations that do. These can include lifting one leg and one arm in the air, and then alternating them.

The main advantage of these core exercises is that you can do them anytime anywhere. You do not need a gym or any equipment. So, if you have a few extra minutes anywhere in your day to do them, go for it!

*there is conflicting evidence regarding the optimal time. Some studies suggest as little as 10 seconds is enough, others suggest 2 minutes, but most agree that longer than 2 minutes does not provide any additional benefit.

Exercises you should never do

The following exercises are considered exercise you should never do, because there is an increased risk of injury without any benefit over some of the exercises shown above.

- Behind the back barbell press, behind the neck pull downs, behind the back pull ups, behind the back anything: this will risk shoulder joint (rotator cuff) injury, and is no better than the exercises done in front of your face.
- Upright barbell row: In this exercise you stand and pull a barbell from your waist height to your chest height. This is another exercise that risks injury to your shoulder joints. The movement impinges (pinches) a tendon between your bone until it weakens. You may not feel pain before the tendon suddenly tears one day.

- Decline bench press: there is no benefit to the chest compared to the flat bench press, and it will give you even less of a workout to the upper pecs.
- Smith machine squat: The Smith machine is a barbell that goes up and down along a fixed track. When the bar is fixed along a track, you are more likely to create uneven stress on your back and knees. In fact, there is probably no good exercise to do on the Smith machine.
- Abdominal crunch machines: abdominal crunches without a machine must be done with good form to prevent stress on your back and neck. Having a machine only increases the chance of improper form and stress.
- Back extensions

Summary of the Program

Once again, here is the program presented again, in case you are still confused about the details.

1. Start your week (or 9 day period) with Workout 1, which involves a lot of heavy barbell or dumbbell lifting: legs, back, chest, and shoulders. For each exercise, start with a light set x 12 - 15 reps, a medium set x 12 reps, and 3 heavy sets of 8 - 12 reps each. For the heavy sets, if you can do more than 12 reps, increase the weight. If you cannot do 8 reps, lighten the weight.

2. If you have some more time at the end of Workout 1, or can fit in an extra workout the very next day, add in an X tra workout focusing on whatever muscle group you would like to. For most people this will probably mean working on the calves and arms (shoulders, biceps, triceps). Once again, for each exercise, start with a light set x 12 - 15 reps, a medium set x 12 reps, and 3 heavy sets of 8 - 12 reps each. For the heavy sets, if you can do more than 12 reps, increase the weight. If you cannot do

8 reps, lighten the weight.

3. Give your muscles at least a day and a half, but preferably 2 days or more, to recover.

4. After enough rest and when your muscles are not sore, but before the week is over, do Workout 2. Choose one exercise for your legs, one for your back, one for your chest, and one for your shoulders. Dumbbells and free weights will give you a better workout than machines. Body weight exercises and band exercises are acceptable as well, but you may need a machine assist or to add weights to stay in the 8 to 12 rep range. Once again, for each exercise, start with a light set x 12 - 15 reps, a medium set x 12 reps, and 3 heavy sets of 8 - 12 reps each. For the heavy sets, if you can do more than 12 reps, increase the weight. If you cannot do 8 reps, lighten the weight.

5. If you didn't do an X-tra workout after Workout 1, then you can do an X-tra workout after Workout 2 instead. It can be on the same day or the very next day. If you don't manage to fit in any X-tra workouts during the week, do not worry. They are not as important as Workout 1 or Workout 2.

6. During your workouts, always remember to focus on form and full range of motion. Raise and lower weights slowly. If you cannot maintain good form, reduce the weight. Rest 2 to 5 minutes between each set.

7. Any time during the week, try to fit in two or three aerobic/cardio sessions. They can be short (10min) and high intensity, or they can be longer (30min) and medium intensity. It does not matter when you do them, although you may find it challenging to do when your legs are very sore from doing barbell squats.

Miscellaneous Questions at the End of the Book (Chapter 11)

- How to choose a gym?
- Is there gym and weight room etiquette?
- How to improve grip strength?
- What to do if you are not improving?
- What about supersets or alternating muscle groups?
- Isn't this a strength training workout over a muscle building one?

Citations

1. Lopes JSS, Machado AF, Micheletti JK, de Almeida AC, Cavina AP, Pastre CM. Effects of training with elastic resistance versus conventional resistance on muscular strength: A systematic review and meta-analysis. *SAGE Open Med*. 2019;7:2050312119831116. Published 2019 Feb 19. doi:10.1177/2050312119831116

2. Bergquist R, Iversen VM, Mork PJ, Fimland MS. Muscle Activity in Upper-Body Single-Joint Resistance Exercises with Elastic Resistance Bands vs. Free Weights. *J Hum Kinet*. 2018;61:5-13. Published 2018 Mar 23. doi:10.1515/hukin-2017-0137

3. Schoenfeld BJ, Ogborn D, Krieger JW. Dose-response relationship between weekly resistance training volume and increases in muscle mass: A systematic review and meta-analysis. *J Sports Sci*. 2017;35(11):1073-1082. doi:10.1080/02640414.2016.1210197

4. Senna G, Scudese E, Martins CL, Scartoni FR, Carneiro F, Camargo Alves JC, Zarlotti C, Martin Dantas EH. Rest Period Length Manipulation on Repetition Consistency for Distinct Single-Joint Exercises *J of*

Exercise Physiol online October 2016 Volume 19 Number 5

Other References

1. Amirthalingam T, Mavros Y, Wilson GC, Clarke JL, Mitchell L, Hackett DA. Effects of a Modified German Volume Training Program on Muscular Hypertrophy and Strength. *J Strength Cond Res*. 2017;31(11):3109-3119. doi:10.1519/JSC.0000000000001747

2. Radaelli R, Fleck SJ, Leite T, et al. Dose-response of 1, 3, and 5 sets of resistance exercise on strength, local muscular endurance, and hypertrophy. *J Strength Cond Res*. 2015;29(5):1349-1358. doi:10.1519/JSC.0000000000000758

3. Schoenfeld BJ. The mechanisms of muscle hypertrophy and their application to resistance training. *J Strength Cond Res*. 2010;24(10):2857-2872. doi:10.1519/JSC.0b013e3181e840f3

4. Schoenfeld BJ, Peterson MD, Ogborn D, Contreras B, Sonmez GT. Effects of Low- vs. High-Load Resistance Training on Muscle Strength and Hypertrophy in Well-Trained Men. *J Strength Cond Res*. 2015;29(10):2954-2963. doi:10.1519/JSC.0000000000000958

5. Schoenfeld BJ, Contreras B, Krieger J, et al. Resistance Training Volume Enhances Muscle Hypertrophy but Not Strength in Trained Men. *Med Sci Sports Exerc*. 2019;51(1):94-103. doi:10.1249/MSS.0000000000001764

6. Wernbom M, Augustsson J, Thomeé R. The influence of frequency, intensity, volume and mode of strength training on whole muscle cross-sectional area in humans. *Sports Med*. 2007;37(3):225-264. doi:10.2165/00007256-200737030-00004

7. Wirth K, Keiner M, Hartmann H, Sander A, Mickel C.

Effect of 8 weeks of free-weight and machine-based strength training on strength and power performance. *J Hum Kinet*. 2016;53:201-210. Published 2016 Oct 15. doi:10.1515/hukin-2016-0023

Chap 5. Aerobic activity and fitness

HIIT versus steady pace

There is a lot of hype about the benefits of high intensity interval training, known as HIIT. HIIT refers to any variation of exercise where you vary the intensity of your workout from very low (or rest) to very high every 30 secs to every few minutes, for usually a total of 10 to 30 minutes. It can mean walking alternating with running as fast as possible, or biking on very low resistance followed by biking on a very high resistance. It can mean doing burpees or jumping rope for one minute followed by one minute of rest. Compared to doing the same aerobic exercise at a steady pace, HIIT has become very popular for the following reasons:

1. You can burn more calories in a shorter period of time. For example, a 20 min HIIT workout on the bike may burn as many calories as a 30min steady pace work out.
2. There is a greater "afterburn" effect, which means your body remains revved up for hours afterwards, thereby "boosting your metabolism"
3. It may promote more type 2 muscle growth because it requires more explosive force against resistance, like weights. Once again, think of a sprinters body compared to a long-distance runner.

Although all of the above is true, the extra calorie burn can be pretty small compared to a steady pace workout. For example, doing a HIIT workout instead of a steady pace workout over 30 minutes might burn 50 more calories during the workout, and perhaps an extra 6 calories / hour over the next 4 to 5 hours (30 more calories), which translates to about the number of calories in a slice of bread. Decreasing the amount of calories you eat will have much more impact than whether you do a HIIT workout vs a steady pace work out.

So, my recommendation is to do what you are most likely to be willing to do.

If you enjoy the challenge of a HIIT workout, go for it. In my experience, most people hate doing them, they can be more stressful on your joints, and are more likely to injure you. So, choose an aerobic workout you can see yourself doing. But whatever you choose, always try to increase the intensity (or length) as you improve. Ideally if you do a steady pace workout, you still want to choose an intensity that makes it difficult to talk and increases your heart rate.

There are many types of exercises that will fall into this category. They can be on machines like a stationary bike, elliptical, treadmill, stationary bike, rowing machine, and many others. They can involve outdoor activities like running, biking, or swimming. They can involve sports like playing basketball or tennis. If going to the gym to do the weight exercises is already an inconvenience, then choose an aerobic activity you can do at home or in your neighborhood or at work. As mentioned before, HIIT exercises may have a slight advantage in calories burned, muscle growth, and improved conditioning but they can also lead to more fatigue and discomfort.

Ultimately the best aerobic exercise is the one you are most likely to do

If you have only 10 minutes, try a HIIT type of exercise.

If you have 30 minutes, choose any activity that you can realistically do for 30 minutes.

Activity for fat loss: Use a fitness tracker.

The main benefit of 10 to 30 minutes of aerobic exercise two to three times a week is to improve your cardiovascular fitness. As you improve your heart and lung conditioning and therefore oxygen delivery to your body, this will allow you to improve your performance in all your activity, including your weight training. It will also improve the efficiency of your type 1 slow fibers. If you really push yourself with some forms of HIIT (step ups, burpees, etc.) you may end up improving type 2 fibers as well.

Unfortunately, aerobic activity 2 to 3 times a week is not enough for help with fat loss. A 180lb person running a 10 minute mile for 30 minutes (3 miles) will burn about 400 calories. Even if there is a slight bump in your metabolism for an hour or two after, it is very small. This certainly can help a bit with fat loss, but you can see that doing this twice a week is not going to compensate for the calories you get eating three meals a day. For that you will have to maintain a high level of activity every day.

Exercise refers to an activity you do specifically to improve your health and fitness. Activity refers to a movement you do for any purpose: walking your dog, going on a hike, pushing a cart while grocery shopping, or cleaning your house. Exercise is a type of activity, but not all activity is considered exercise. When it comes to using energy, your body does not know the difference between activity and exercise. Your body only knows movement and that it needs to use energy to move. You should consider activity as a form of exercise as well, as long as you can measure it.

If you are more interested in losing fat than gaining muscle (or want to be extra sure you do not gain fat), you will need to be active throughout the day. A rough rule of thumb is that walking at a moderate to brisk pace (3.0 to 3.5 miles per hour) for 30 minutes will burn about 1 calorie for every pound of body weight. In other words, a 180 lb. person walking briskly for 30 minutes may burn about 180 calories. This may seem a bit depressing, but that same person may only burn about 40 - 50 calories sitting. So, getting out of your chair and walking can essentially triple or quadruple your "metabolism" and the amount of calories you burn. **In other words, low intensity is way better than no intensity.** Ultimately what may limit you is not your ability, but the hours in your day and all your other responsibilities. For this reason, if you are trying to lose fat, I strongly recommend a fitness tracker (clip on, bracelet type, or watch) to motivate you to get the maximum number of steps a day. If possible, aim for 10,000 steps a day or more. This is roughly 5 miles. Assuming you are paying attention to how you are eating, keeping your body moving throughout the day is essential if you want to maintain a calorie deficit, AND you want to avoid the metabolic adaptation (drop in your metabolism) that occurs when you eat less. Because a fitness tracker monitors your activity like an exercise, you can now consider every activity as a form of exercise.

Measuring Progress

Just like your resistance workouts, you want to be able to measure your aerobic ability in some way. Most aerobic workouts involve some combination of time, distance, speed (distance over time), or calories burned. Usually, you will keep either time OR distance the same for each workout, and measure your improvement in the other variable.

For example, if you decide to run or bike 20 minutes every workout, you will measure how far you travel (or how far your machine says you travel) with each workout. As you improve, your total distance (and average speed) will increase. If you are using an exercise machine that calculates calories, your total calories used will also increase. Please remember, these calories are based on a mathematical equation of work needed to use the machine, and may be very different than the actual calories your body burns.

Alternatively, you can decide that you always want to travel a certain distance. As you improve, the time it takes you to complete the distance will decrease. And hence, your speed will increase. A common way to measure your running ability is to calculate your average time to run one mile.

Don't Worry About Heart Rate

There are a lot of studies about how getting to certain target heart rates are needed to achieve the most cardiovascular benefit. Although this is true, using heart rate as a measure of your exercise is rarely practical. There is always some benefit to movement whether you hit your target heart rate with each workout or not. If you measure your overall progress, and try to improve over time, your exercise tolerance and heart health will automatically improve.

Summary

1. Do some type of aerobic (cardiovascular) activity twice a week or more. You can choose longer (30minutes) with moderate intensity, or shorter (10-20 minutes) with high intensity. The differences between HIIT workouts and moderate intensity workouts are not that significant.

2. Ultimately the most important thing is to choose an aerobic activity that you enjoy doing (or at least learn to enjoy).

3. Moderate and high intensity workouts will help your cardiovascular fitness and endurance, which improves your overall health and physical ability.

4. If you are trying to lose fat or want to have some extra insurance against gaining fat, you must move as much as possible throughout the day. Use a fitness tracker to remind you to move and measure your daily movement. Aim for a daily average of 10,000 steps or 5 miles.

References

1. DeFina LF, Radford NB, Barlow CE, et al. Association of All-Cause and Cardiovascular Mortality With High Levels of Physical Activity and Concurrent Coronary Artery Calcification. *JAMA Cardiol*. 2019;4(2):174-181. doi:10.1001/jamacardio.2018.4628

2. Foster C, Farland CV, Guidotti F, et al. The Effects of High Intensity Interval Training vs Steady State Training on Aerobic and Anaerobic Capacity. *J Sports Sci Med*. 2015;14(4):747-755. Published 2015 Nov 24.

3. Sevits KJ, Melanson EL, Swibas T, et al. Total daily energy expenditure is increased following a single bout of sprint interval training. *Physiol Rep*. 2013;1(5):e00131. doi:10.1002/phy2.131

4. Stokes KA, Nevill ME, Hall GM, Lakomy HK. The time course of the human growth hormone response to a 6 s and a 30 s cycle ergometer sprint. *J Sports Sci*. 2002;20(6):487-494. doi:10.1080/02640410252925152

5. Zhang H, Tong TK, Qiu W, et al. Comparable Effects of High-Intensity Interval Training and Prolonged Continuous Exercise Training on Abdominal Visceral Fat Reduction in Obese Young Women. *J Diabetes Res*. 2017;2017:5071740. doi:10.1155/2017/507174

Chap 6. A diet for the rest of your life

Your "diet"

When people say they are "on a diet" they often mean they are on some type of nutrition plan that is very regimented. Usually, the diet has very specific rules about specific foods, and usually promises to help you lose fat quickly. There are usually enough rules to fill an entire book, which is always a great way to make money. Or instead of rules, they simply create premade meals or recipes or supplements that you have to stick to. Another great way to make money. Most of these diets are short lived, and people cannot maintain them for too long. Once they quit, many people gain back more weight than they started with. Many diets work for a short time by forcing you to increase your awareness of the way you eat, but the rules are too complicated, or too hard to follow lifelong. Other diets have predetermined meals that you must stick to and that require no awareness at all. Over time, the diet does not fit into your regular lifestyle and routine, or cravings give in because you restricted too much too soon, and the diet usually falls apart.

The true definition of the word "diet" is simply "food that a person habitually eats." In other words, your diet really refers to the way you eat regularly, whether you are following a specific plan or not. You may be very aware of your diet or you may be not paying attention to it at all. You may be eating a very healthy diet, or a very unhealthy one. So, your goal is not to go on a "diet", but to develop healthy eating habits that will eventually add up to a healthy lifelong diet.

Your success with weight training and activity is ultimately determined by your drive and mental effort. In the same way, your success with eating healthy is ultimately determined by your awareness. If you want to eat healthier, you do have to remember a few rules around the WHAT you eat, but more importantly you have to increase your awareness of WHY and HOW you eat. For the rest of your life. This allows for a diet that is healthy, realistic, allows for variety, and fits into your lifestyle and the people you eat with. It allows for some super healthy days, and some not so healthy days, but hopefully gets you used to eating healthier overall.

The only diet guidelines you really need to know

Here are the proven guidelines that can improve your long-term health and fitness. I call them guidelines instead of rules, because the word "rules" implies that you must follow them 100% of the time, and leads to an all or nothing mindset which actually sabotages you in the long run. You need to be conscious and aware of these guidelines every time you eat or drink, even if you do not actually follow them 100% of the time. Being conscious and aware also means accurate recording with a calorie counting app or a food log. If you try to be conscious of these guidelines with every meal and follow them 80 to 90% of the time, you will start to improve your health.

Here are the guidelines you need to remember:

1. Minimize sugar, alcohol, and hours. Minimize means eating these items as rarely as possible.
2. Maximize protein and water, and spread them out across the day
3. Avoid processed foods whenever possible
4. Eat mindfully and slowly: treat food as fuel and acknowledge your reason for eating every time you eat. Eat slow enough to notice when you are no longer hungry.

5. Verify your awareness with a calorie counting app or a food log.

Minimize added sugar.

Added sugar (sugar, sucrose, high fructose corn syrup, cane sugar, raw sugar, cane juice, fructose, glucose, sucrose) is the easiest way to get calories from food without having to spend any energy on digestion. It is absorbed from your food into your bloodstream and into your cells very quickly. Because of this, added sugar is associated with weight gain, obesity, diabetes, heart disease, cancer, and a host of other medical problems. (Giugliano,Khan,Choo) There is absolutely no health benefit to sugar except for getting energy quickly when you need it right away during a race or athletic event. If you are going to look at only one ingredient on the label, look at the sugar content and make the following conversion: 4 grams of sugar = 1 teaspoon. That means drinking a can of soda with 39 g of sugar is essentially drinking 9 teaspoons of sugar. Go over to your sugar bowl and put 9 teaspoons of sugar into a glass. Would you ever be willing to eat that much sugar at once? Yet we do every time we have a can or bottle of soda. If you are eating a sugary food like a donut, or cake, or a cookie but you do not have the label, always look it up using a calorie counting app. When you do this, you may be surprised to learn that a glazed Krispy Kreme donut has 10 grams of sugar (2 ½ teaspoons) which is not ideal, but still much less than a glass of orange juice with 22 grams of sugar (5 ½ teaspoons)!

Over time you will eventually memorize the values and no longer need to look them up every time.

In general, the easiest way to minimize sugar in your diet is to minimize drinks with sugar. Most juices, smoothies, shakes, and sodas will have a significant amount of sugar. In addition, drinks pass through your stomach quickly, do not make you feel

...ud usually make you crave even more sugar because of the way your hormones and taste buds respond to them. Try to minimize the sugar in your teas and coffees.

The studies around diet and zero sugar drinks are unclear. Although they do not contain calories related to sugar, most studies suggest that they can trigger similar hormonal responses, increasing your craving for more sugar. I would say that if soda is one of the vices you truly cannot stay away from, and you are trying to lose fat, diet drinks are probably better than sugar drinks, but you have to be even more mindful of the sugars in the food you eat throughout the day. The zero-calorie sugar substitute xylitol is deadly in dogs because it causes a surge in insulin, which drops their blood sugar and leads to seizures. So clearly, even though these sugar substitutes have zero calories, the body can often hormonal responses that are similar to sugar. (Tandel,Mattes)

Natural sugar in fruits is a combination of sucrose, glucose, and fructose. Although chemically they are like added sugars in pure form, fruits have additional nutrients, electrolytes, and fiber that are overall healthy for the body. Fruits take time and work to digest, and because the sugar is not absorbed rapidly into the body, and fructose seems to trigger less of a hormonal response than glucose, you do not get the hormonal responses that lead to diabetes and other medical problems. This is known as having a low glycemic score. Fruit juices on the other hand, have high glycemic scores mainly because they are so rapidly absorbed and require so little work for digestion.

For most people, avoiding foods with added sugar will make a huge difference in their health. If you are ready to take it a step further, or need even better sugar control because of prediabetes or diabetes, then you can try to replace high glycemic foods with low glycemic foods. Treat high glycemic carbohydrates like sugar. These include foods like white bread, potatoes, white rice, instant oatmeal, and many baked goods. Replace them with low glycemic foods like brown rice, whole grain bread, steel cut oatmeal, and fruits whenever possible.

Minimize alcohol

There is no good nutritional value in alcohol. The most recent studies show that there are no significant health benefits to alcohol. (National Inst, GBD 2016) Period. There is always more potential harm than good. The old studies suggesting that red wine or other forms of alcohol are good for the heart were flawed, or showed that the benefits were marginal compared to the downsides. Some studies suggest that there may be mechanisms by which alcohol can lead to either fat gain or difficulty with fat loss due to a variety of factors. Some of these mechanisms may include increased hunger and decreased testosterone, although the evidence is still unclear. Your body always metabolizes alcohol over fat. The benefits of keeping your belly fat down and exercising regularly are far greater than the benefit of any alcoholic drink. Save alcohol for special social occasions, as an addition to a positive experience. Do not drink alone. Do not drink to "relax" or "soothe" yourself at the end of the day. If you cannot find healthier ways to relax or calm yourself, you start to become dependent, and dependence is just a milder form of addiction.

When you do decide to have a celebratory drink, from a strict nutritional perspective, it is probably better to have wine or hard liquor over beer, or a sweet drink made with sugar. Beer has a lower percentage of alcohol and more carbohydrates than higher proof wine or hard liquor.

Minimize the number of hours you eat in the day

Intermittent fasting refers to fasting for as long as possible in a 24-hour day. The most common routines involve limiting all your eating to perhaps 8 hours (i.e., 10am to 6pm) and not eating anything in the remaining 16 hours. You can drink water or zero calorie drinks (i.e., black coffee) any time. There is a lot of interest in intermittent fasting, and the early research is relatively promising. Most studies show multiple benefits: better weight loss, better muscle gain, and improved cholesterol and diabetes. [Patterson] However, studies that suggest decreased cancer risk or longer life are largely based on animals. Also, intermittent fasting usually results in fewer overall calories eaten per day, which may ultimately be more important than the hours themselves. In addition, as in many fads, there may be a bias to publish studies that show a benefit over studies that show no difference.

Intermittent fasting for the rest of your life takes a fair amount of discipline, and also requires you to keep a relatively rigid routine every day. If you live and eat alone, this may be possible, but if you prepare meals and eat with your family, friends, or coworkers, this may not be practical.

My recommendation is to be conscious of when you eat your first and last bite of food every day. You do not have to adhere to intermittent fasting every day for the rest of your life, but on those days you can realistically eat a bit less in the morning or at night, try to do so. If you wake up late on a weekend morning and don't feel too hungry right away, put off eating breakfast a little longer. Or have brunch. If you are bored after dinner and feeling like raiding the refrigerator for some dessert, ask yourself if you really need to. Eating from 7:30 am to 8pm may not technically qualify as intermittent fasting, but it's still better than eating from 7am to 11 pm. That's three hours of food that you didn't need to eat, and given that you aren't exercising afterward, would turn to fat overnight.

Despite the popularity of many intermittent fasting routines that start with a late breakfast, there are many studies that suggest it is better to eat before activity rather than after it. This allows your body to use food you just ate as fuel rather than store it as fat. For most of us who are active during the day, that usually means it is better to have a bigger breakfast and a smaller dinner rather than the other way around. People who barely eat during the day but then have a large high calorie meal just before they go to sleep are usually the most likely to put on fat. If you must choose between skipping breakfast and skipping dessert, definitely skip dessert. Dessert should be for the rare special occasion.

Maximize protein

The "minimum" recommendation for protein is about 0.8 grams of protein per kilogram of body weight per day. This is about 0.36 grams protein per pound of body weight. For a 165lb person, this is about 60 grams of protein a day.

However, when weight training regularly and trying to build muscle, most programs (*and the Am College of Sports Medicine) recommend 1.2 - 1.7 gm per kg of body weight, which is about 0.5 to 0.8 grams per pound. Adults age 50 to 75 preserve more muscle eating 1.5gms per kg body weight than those eating 0.8 grams. High performance athletes and those trying to gain muscle as rapidly as possible may need to take in 1.6 to 2.0 gms of protein per kg of body weight. (Jager, Schoenfeld) Except for someone with known kidney disease, there is no known downside to consuming too much protein.

If you are overweight, and have a lot of fat, use your lean body weight instead of your total weight. If you truly know your total body fat, your lean body weight is what's left over. For example, if you know you are at 25% body fat, and weigh 250lbs, then your lean body weight is 250 lbs. x 75% which is around 190lbs.

An easier way is to just guess by imagining how much you would weigh if you get to your goal body. For example, if you are a 250lb person who is aiming to lose more fat and gain enough muscle to look somewhat athletic, you might guesstimate that you might realistically end up at 210lbs. You can use this number for your calculations.

Let's summarize the recommendations:

Grams Protein	grams/ kg/day	grams/ lb./day	125l b	150lb	175lb	200lb	225lb lean
Minimum	0.8	0.4	50	54	63	72	82
Medium performanc e/growth	1.5	0.7	88	102	118	135	153
High performanc e/growth	2.0	0.9	113	136	158	180	204

In general, you should aim for the medium performance and muscle growth range of about 0.7 grams/ pound. To make the calculation easier, you can increase it to about 0.75, and say **you should eat at least about 1 gram of protein per lb. x 75% (or ¾) of your body weight.** If you eat more, it may sometimes be better, and will not be harmful.

Having a lot of protein is not enough. You have to aim to keep the percent of protein in your diet high, which means taking a lot of protein without increasing your carbohydrates or fats at the same time. The literature for this type of diet is overwhelmingly positive. (Arentson,Kim, Leidy) Dietary guidelines recommend getting 10 to 35% of your calories from protein. Aiming for closer to 35% provides for better muscle preservation and growth, decreases the chance of diabetes, and prevents overeating. If you are on a higher calorie diet to gain muscle, sticking to a higher percent protein diet will also minimize the extra fat you gain. So, this is where food choices start to make a big difference, because getting to 35% of your total calories from protein is much harder than it seems. But when you aim for this, the fat and carbs will automatically be kept to low and healthy levels.

Let's look at how many calories come from protein in some common foods. The numbers below are ballpark numbers, since they can vary by brand or preparation. In the chart below, if a food has 50% protein calories, that means that the other 50% of the calories in that food come from carbohydrates or fats. If you are interested in foods not mentioned below, look on the internet under "caloric ratio tool". Do not confuse the numbers below with the % recommended daily allowance numbers you may see on the food label. The % RDA numbers are based on what they consider the recommended diet for the "average" person, but there really is no such thing, and the % RDA numbers are not really meaningful.

FOOD	% Calories from Protein
Canned tuna in water	80-94%
Protein supplements, shakes	70-90%
Cooked shrimp (plain)	90%
Chicken breast no skin	80%
Turkey breast	80-85%

Cottage cheese	59%-69%
Greek yogurt full fat	30%
Greek yogurt 0% fat	75%
Lean beef	53%
Salmon: sockeye	60%
Salmon: wild Atlantic	55%
Salmon: farmed Atlantic	40%
Nonfat no sugar Greek yogurt	48%
Large egg	35%
Whole milk	21%
Broccoli	20%-30%
Soy milk	16%
Quinoa	15%
Oats	15%
Almonds	15%
Almond milk	4%
Brown rice	7%

When you look at the foods above you can see why bodybuilders and actors trying to get big will spend their days eating chicken breast, wild (not farmed) salmon, cottage cheese, and protein supplements, to keep their overall protein percentage high. For vegetables and carbs, they choose high protein carbs like broccoli, quinoa, and brown rice.

Eating beef will give you lots of protein, but over 45% of the other calories are still coming from fat. Eating eggs will give you lots of protein, but 65% of the calories are still coming from fats and carbs. And almonds still have way more fat calories than protein calories. And almond milk essentially has no protein, even though it comes from almonds.

When you look at the percentages above, you can see why trying to get 10 to 35% of your total calories from protein is actually quite difficult. With the exception of lean chicken breast, canned tuna, and shrimp, even the foods that we consider "proteins" still give us lots of calories from fats and carbs. Once you add other fats and carbs to your diet, as you should, the total percentage of calories from protein drops down even further.

The following screenshots are examples of the graphs a common calorie counting app will show you. Almost all the calorie counting apps should be able to show you your total protein intake in grams, and as a percentage of the total calories eaten that day. **Try to get at least 10-35% of your total calories from protein. When you are trying to build muscle, try to make sure you are eating at least 1 gram of protein x 75% (or ¾) of your body weight (in pounds).** Once you enter your food into one of these apps, you can get a great sense of both numbers.

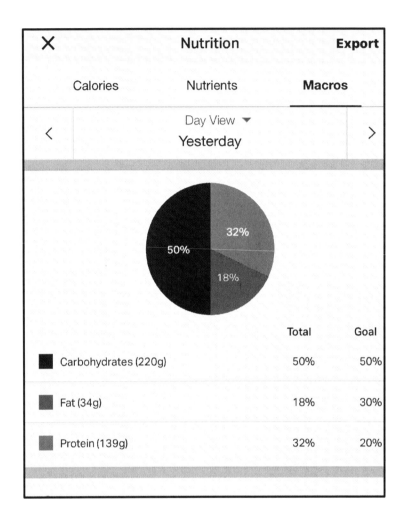

	Total	Goal
Carbohydrates (220g)	50%	50%
Fat (34g)	18%	30%
Protein (139g)	32%	20%

	Calories	**Nutrients**	Macros

Day View ▼

< Yesterday >

	Total	Goal	Left
Protein	140	113	-27g ›
Carbohydrates	221	283	62g ›
Fiber	19	30	11g ›
Sugar	71	85	14g ›
Fat	35	75	40g ›
Saturated Fat	6	25	19g ›
Polyunsaturated Fat	2	-	-2g ›
Monounsaturated Fat	6	-	-6g ›
Trans Fat	0	0	0g ›

Protein supplements

Protein shakes can be very helpful when your goal is to get as much protein as possible without getting additional calories from fat or sugar. They are convenient and easy to drink on the go. If you are on a purely plant-based diet or minimizing meat and dairy, they are also a good way to make sure you are getting enough essential amino acids.

Choosing the right shake:
Choose one with as much protein as possible (at least 40 grams per drink) and with as little sugar and fat as possible, that still tastes good enough for you to drink regularly. Make sure you choose a drink that is specifically intended to be a protein supplement (i.e., Isopure, muscle milk, etc.) and not a nutritional supplement (i.e., Ensure, Boost, etc.) which have a lot of fat and carbohydrates. When you enter your shake into a calorie counting app, it should show that at least 80% of the calories come from protein. If you don't mind the taste of one that is 90% or more, even better. There is a lot of debate about the different forms of protein used in the various shakes: dairy (whey, casein, milk) and plant-based (soy, pea, rice, etc.). In general whey protein is absorbed the fastest, and may lead to the best recovery taken right after workouts, but there are no convincing studies to prove this leads to better results for the average athlete. Most people will usually try a few different brands before they decide on one they like, or can at least tolerate. The powder forms are cheaper per gram protein than the premade prepackaged drinks.

Most men should try to avoid soy drinks because they contain estrogens that can worsen or lead to gynecomastia ("man boobs").

When should you take protein shakes?
There are many studies looking at the timing of protein shakes on muscle growth and strength, and ultimately there may be a slight advantage to taking whey shakes within 2 hours after workouts, but the advantage is probably negligible. There are

other studies that recommend taking protein just prior to bed. Ultimately the most important factor is getting enough protein into your body whenever your muscle is trying to repair itself, which means throughout the day. This means, in addition to the protein shake, try to distribute the amount of protein you eat across all your meals. In reality, that is the only way you can realistically even hope to approach getting 20% or more of your calories from protein.

I recommend at minimum a protein shake on the day of any weight workout (preferably after the workout) and the day after. After two days, if your muscles are still sore, assume your muscles are trying to recover and rebuild, and take one on those days as well. If your aerobic workouts also lead to muscle soreness, do the same for them. **In other words, when you are working out fairly frequently, take at least one protein shake (40gm or more) daily to help you get to your medium performance protein goal (1 gram of protein x 75% of your body weight in pounds). When you are working out less frequently, take a protein shake on the day of your workout, the day after, and every day your muscles feel sore.**

Maximize water
Staying hydrated allows your cells and body to perform at their highest level. Dehydration can impair both brain function and metabolism.   Every study supports the idea that hydration improves performance, and dehydration impairs it. If you are someone who sweats easily or breathes heavily, you may be particularly sensitive to dehydration. If you are good at measuring everything you eat and drink, the recommended amount of water each day is roughly 8 glasses of 8 oz each = 64oz total.   Another way to make sure you are hydrated throughout the day is making sure your urine is relatively pale

and not dark yellow. Try to stay hydrated throughout the day and especially during your workout.

All drinks, and even food, contain water, so it is okay to count all your drinks throughout the day, including the amount of water you add to your protein shake. Although drinking soda or other sugary drinks is still hydrating, you should avoid them since you are trying to minimize sugar. Remember, 4 grams of sugar = 1 teaspoon. Although some people will tell you that drinking coffee will dehydrate you, this is really not true. So as long as you do not add sugar, you can include your cups of coffee into your water total.

Avoid Processed Foods

As noted in Chapter 3, there are many studies that consistently show processed foods are more likely to lead to weight gain. Processed meats particularly have been linked to heart disease, high blood pressure, and other diseases. There are multiple theories for this. In addition to the high salts, chemicals, and preservatives used in processed foods, there is something about actually processing the foods that breaks down the food molecules and makes them easier to digest and absorb into the bloodstream. This means processed foods require less energy to break down, which means more calories absorbed into your body in a shorter amount of time. This means you are more likely to get more calories from the food, and feel hungry again sooner.

Meat vs Plant based diets

There is a lot of conflicting and confusing research on plant-based diets versus meat-based diets. It is clear that a purely plant-based diet is associated with better health and a longer life than a diet that includes a lot of red meat. It is clear that a diet with a lot of red meat will increase the risk of heart disease, stroke, and early death. However, it is not clear that a strictly plant-based diet like a vegan diet is healthier than a diet that includes lean meats or fish. It becomes even more confusing because some of the research allows plant-based diets to include fish, which really isn't plant based. Another area of confusion is that the nutritional definition of red meat includes all mammals (beef, veal, mutton, lamb, pork, venison, rabbit, etc.) while culinary definitions may consider veal, lamb, rabbit, and some cuts of pork as white meat.

We can order the diets from most restrictive to least restrictive in the following way:

1. Plant based only (vegan)
2. Above, dairy allowed
3. Above, fish allowed
4. Above, white meat poultry allowed
5. Above, all poultry allowed
6. Above, red meat and processed meat allowed

Assuming you avoid processed foods and sugar, then most likely the red meat heavy diet will have a higher risk of heart disease and being overweight, while the vegan diet will have the least. Of course, it is also important to get enough protein to maintain muscle mass and health, which is completely possible with a vegan diet but requires much more attention to finding vegan proteins that will give you enough of the nine essential amino acids. When we look at the areas of the world with the longest lifespan known as Blue Zones (Sardinia in Italy, Okinawa in Japan, Nicoya in Costa Rica, etc.) we find that most people have a simple largely plant based diet supplemented occasionally with lean meat or fish. However, these populations also lead a very active lifestyle moving throughout the day, tend to eat larger meals in the morning rather than the evening, and eat to "80% full". The saying in Okinawa is "Hara Hachi Bu."

If you want to follow a strict 100% plant-based diet for ethical reasons related to the treatment of animals, I understand. However, from a strictly nutritional perspective, you do not have to eliminate red meat, processed meat, or a certain type of meat for the rest of your life. Instead, try to make eating red meat a rare occurrence, and on most days try to get your protein from the healthier choices. If you are celebrating with friends with a steak dinner, go for it. But on a routine basis, try to get your protein from white meat, fish, and dairy. If you can get good protein from plant-based foods, then you do not have to eat white meat, fish, or dairy every single day. On the other hand, there is no definitive study to suggest you are worse off if you do have lean white meat or fish every day. If you truly enjoy a vegetarian (dairy allowed) or vegan diet (no dairy allowed) and can see yourself eating that way lifelong, just make sure you are getting enough protein.

And as the "80% full" mentality suggests, how you eat is just as important as what you eat.

Calorie counting

Ultimately your ability to gain muscle or lose fat is going to depend on the type of food AND on the total number of calories you eat every day. If you want to gain muscle, you must eat more calories than you use. If you want to lose fat, you must eat less calories than you use.

As we age, we do not need as many calories per day as we thought. The Mayo Clinic healthy weight calorie counter (google it for latest website) suggests that the average 40 year old woman only needs 1400-1700 calories a day, and the average 40 year old man only needs 1900 to 2100 calories a day.

If they absorb more than this into their bloodstream and into their cells, they will need to use up the extra energy for activity in order to not gain weight.

How many calories a day should you aim for? It depends on multiple factors and your goals, and I will explain how you determine what to aim for in the next chapter. However, no matter what number you aim for, you must use calorie counting and food journaling on some level to improve your understanding of food and your individual habits. The vast majority of people have very little awareness of what and how much then eat every day, and most people underestimate the total volume and calories they eat each day. When they actually enter everything they eat in the calorie counting app, they are usually surprised at the result.

Here is what you need to do:
1. Get a calorie counting app on your smartphone and start using it now. It is tedious and time consuming entering foods in the beginning. Over time, as you save your favorites and most popular foods, it becomes easier to use. It is easier to know the calories in your food today than it has ever been. The only irony is that processed packaged foods (which are unhealthy) are easier to enter than foods you cook from scratch (which are healthier). Homemade cooking is harder to enter in because you either have to put in every single ingredient individually, or you have to approximate using the generic versions of foods already found in the apps.
2. You do not have to use a calorie counting app every day for the rest of your life, but use it frequently enough that you start to memorize the calories and sugar content and protein content in the foods you eat.
3. We tend to use calorie counting apps when we are trying

to "eat healthy" but it is especially important to use them during periods when we know we are not eating healthy. This is where you can really learn which particular foods sabotage your goals the most.

4. Make sure to enter everything you eat. Don't forget little bites or snacks you may forget about later. If you don't have time to enter something in the moment, take a picture with your phone and enter it at the end of the day.

5. It is okay to guesstimate. You do not have to be too accurate. Even when you find the right food to enter, entering the exact portion size can be confusing. Do your best. It is okay as long as your guesstimates are relatively consistent, because as I will explain in the next chapter, the accuracy of calories is not that important. What is important is that you have some type of number to establish a baseline which you will then either decrease or increase depending on your goals.

6. Meat is easiest to measure in oz. 1 pound is 16 oz. So, 4 oz of meat is a ¼ pound. Fruits and vegetables are easiest to guesstimate by volume: ½ cup, 1 cup, etc. For fluids, 8 fluid oz. is one cup. 32 fluid oz. is 4 cups which is 1 quart.

7. At the end of every day, look at the total number of calories (your target depends on your goals in Chap 7), the total grams of sugar (as little as possible), the total grams of protein (aim for 1 gram of protein for 75% of your weight in pounds), and the percent of calories you got from protein (10 to 35%). At the end of each week look at your weekly average.

Mindful and Slow eating

Studies show that when given a bowl of all brown M and M's instead of colored M and M's, they tend to eat much fewer M and M's. So clearly there are factors that we are not even aware of that influence how we eat.

If you are reading this, you are probably not struggling to find your next meal, or going hungry for days. You probably have food easily available whenever you want it. So ultimately, it is your brain that determines when you eat, what you eat, and how you eat. Training your brain is the most important part of eating healthy for the rest of your life.

The best way to ultimately control how you eat is to increase your awareness around food and eating, and to be mindful of this every single time you eat. Even if you eat a piece of candy, or cake, or drink some soda, you at least acknowledge that you aren't making a very healthy choice, and you know (hopefully) that it is a rare occurrence and the exception rather than the rule.

1. Before any first bite (or sip), ask yourself if you are eating for energy. If not, ask yourself why you are eating, and if you really need to. Here are some examples of eating when we really do not need to
   - ❑ Bored. (nothing to do, raid the cupboard or refrigerator to munch on something
   - ❑ Social (a party, BBQ, celebration dinner, etc.)
   - ❑ Entertainment (movie popcorn or candy, food at a sporting event or show, etc.)
   - ❑ Reward (an ice cream with your kids, a drink after a hard day's work)
   - ❑ Soothing emotions or stress (a bowl of ice cream or a drink help dull uncomfortable emotions)
   - ❑ Chance. The food happened to be there. (coworkers bring in food, somebody else is eating a snack, etc.)

❑ Cravings and pleasure. Is a craving the same as hunger, or is it a desire or thought for a food you think will bring you pleasure?

❑ Stress, fatigue, anxiety

❑ If you eat frequently for some of the reasons above, breaking these habits can be very difficult, but calling out these habits into your consciousness and awareness is the first step. Pausing before your first bite and recognizing the reason for eating will increase your willpower over time.

2. Eat as slowly as possible and stop when you are no longer hungry. Chew your food slowly, savor the taste, and pay attention to how you are eating. Pause as long as possible between bites. It may take 15 min for signals from the stomach to let the brain know it is full. Pausing between bites allows you to realize you may be close to full before you are. You do not need to eat until you are full or uncomfortable. You only need to eat until you are no longer hungry. Hence the expression "Hara Hachi Bu", or "eat until you are 80% full."

3. Avoid distractions. People eat more when watching TV, surfing the internet, or talking with friends.

4. Break the habit of having to eat everything on the plate. If you are trying to eat less (it depends on your goals in Chap 7), use small plates.

Avoid All or Nothing Thinking

If you follow the guidelines most of the time, you will find it easier and easier to follow them over time. If you have some food with a lot of sugar, or have some alcohol, simply acknowledge this to yourself and accept it. At the end of the month, you should have an accurate idea of how often you did not follow the guidelines. Was it 5% of the time? 10%? 20%? If you have no idea, try to do a better job logging your food in your calorie counting app or food journal. Try to find the balance where you follow the guidelines most of the time, but can still indulge yourself with some sugar or alcohol occasionally without feeling guilty or like a failure.

In 2016, on the Tonight show, Dwayne "the Rock" Johnson claimed he had not eaten a single piece of candy in 27 years. There are ultra-disciplined people like the Rock. But most of us start to feel deprived when we go to those extremes. Often, when we try to follow "rules" 100% of the time, we either become overly obsessive about them, or start to crave the foods we can no longer have. These cravings are more mental than physical. Ultimately, when we "give in" to these cravings, we feel like we have failed or broken the "rules", and we rightfully conclude that it will be impossible to follow these rules lifelong. This conclusion, along with the shame of giving in to cravings, usually convinces us to abandon the entire diet completely. This is why people who try to lose weight too quickly often "yo-yo" and regain all or more of their weight back. They go "all in" to lose weight as quickly as possible, but eventually find the rules too hard to follow 100% of the time, and then give up completely.

Try to avoid this "all or nothing" thinking. Your goal is to eat healthy most of the time, but not all of the time. That is the only way most of us can maintain a truly healthy diet for the next 10, 20, or 50 years.

Any other guidelines?

If you have the willpower to eat even "healthier" than the diet I have suggested, feel free to proceed as long as you feel fairly confident you can maintain your choices lifelong. So, if you truly have the willpower, what would eating "healthier" look like?

- Choose protein from mainly fish and legumes (beans, peas, lentils, soybeans) which is the basis for most Mediterranean and "blue zone" diets.
- Eat only whole grain and low glycemic carbs.
- Try to increase Omega -3 (a type of polyunsaturated fat) as much as possible. The most health promoting forms of Omega-3 come from fish. Flax seeds, walnuts, canola oil, and soybean oil also have Omega-3, but they must be converted by the body from the plant type to the fish type of Omega-3, and it is not very efficient, and probably not enough.
- Minimize saturated fats as much as possible, but don't substitute them with high glycemic carbs. Saturated fat is found in cheese, pizza, milk, butter, dairy, red meat, processed meat, and most fast foods.
- Replace your saturated fats with more monounsaturated fats. Monounsaturated fats include olive oil, peanut oil, canola oil, avocados, many nuts, pumpkin seeds, sesame seeds, and other types of nuts and seeds.
- Eliminate all trans fats, which is a processed fat found in margarines, shortening, and many processed foods. Luckily most packaged foods have tried to eliminate trans-fat in their ingredients.

Summary: Putting it all together

1. Decide your priority: Do you need a calorie deficit to help with fat loss, or a calorie surplus to help with muscle gain? (see the next chapter)
2. Minimize sugar, alcohol, processed foods, and the hours you eat (especially happy hour and desert hour).
3. Maximize protein. If you are trying to gain muscle, aim for AT LEAST the medium performance growth range,

which is 1 gram of protein x 75% of your body weight in pounds. More protein is safe, unless you have known kidney disease. You should get 10 to 35% of your total calories from protein. Use your calorie counting app to verify both numbers.

4. Maximize your water. You should feel hydrated and your urine should be very light.

5. Use protein supplements (40g or more) on workout days, the day after a workout, and any day your muscles feel tired or sore. If you are exercising 4 to 7 days a week, then just take one every day.

6. Start using a calorie counting app. Count your total calories, and the percent of calories that come from protein. Count your total grams of sugar, and your total grams of protein.

7. Be mindful: eat for energy, and minimize eating for other reasons. Eat slowly. Stop eating when you are no longer hungry.

8. Do not try to be perfect and avoid "all or nothing" thinking.

9. Continuously measure progress and continuously adjust. Do not quit when you do not see results quickly. (see next chapter)

Citations

1. Giugliano D, Maiorino MI, Bellastella G, Esposito K. More sugar? No, thank you! The elusive nature of low carbohydrate diets. *Endocrine*. 2018;61(3):383-387. doi:10.1007/s12020-018-1580-x

2. Khan TA, Sievenpiper JL. Controversies about sugars: results from systematic reviews and meta-analyses on obesity, cardiometabolic disease and diabetes. *Eur J Nutr*. 2016;55(Suppl 2):25-43. doi:10.1007/s00394-016-1345-3

3. Choo VL, Viguiliouk E, Blanco Mejia S, et al. Food sources of fructose-containing sugars and glycaemic control: systematic review and meta-analysis of controlled intervention studies [published correction appears in BMJ. 2019 Oct 9;367:l5524]. BMJ. 2018;363:k4644. Published 2018 Nov 21. doi:10.1136/bmj.k4644

4. Tandel KR. Sugar substitutes: Health controversy over perceived benefits. *J Pharmacol Pharmacother.* 2011;2(4):236-243. doi:10.4103/0976-500X.85936

5. Mattes RD, Popkin BM. Nonnutritive sweetener consumption in humans: effects on appetite and food intake and their putative mechanisms. *Am J Clin Nutr.* 2009;89(1):1-14. doi:10.3945/ajcn.2008.26792

6. National Institute on Alcohol Abuse and Alcoholism: Alcohol facts and statistics.

7. GBD 2016 Alcohol Collaborators. Alcohol use and burden for 195 countries and territories, 1990-2016: a systematic analysis for the Global Burden of Disease Study 2016 [published correction appears in Lancet. 2018 Sep 29;392(10153):1116] [published correction appears in Lancet. 2019 Jun 22;393(10190):e44]. *Lancet.* 2018;392(10152):1015-1035. doi:10.1016/S0140-6736(18)31310-2

8. Patterson RE, Laughlin GA, LaCroix AZ, et al. Intermittent Fasting and Human Metabolic Health. *J Acad Nutr Diet.* 2015;115(8):1203-1212. doi:10.1016/j.jand.2015.02.018

9. Jäger R, Kerksick CM, Campbell BI, et al. International Society of Sports Nutrition Position Stand: protein and exercise. *J Int Soc Sports Nutr.* 2017;14:20. Published 2017 Jun 20. doi:10.1186/s12970-017-0177-8

10. Schoenfeld BJ, Aragon AA, Krieger JW. The effect of protein timing on muscle strength and hypertrophy: a

meta-analysis. *J Int Soc Sports Nutr.* 2013;10(1):53. Published 2013 Dec 3. doi:10.1186/1550-2783-10-53

11. Arentson-Lantz E, Clairmont S, Paddon-Jones D, Tremblay A, Elango R. Protein: A nutrient in focus. *Appl Physiol Nutr Metab.* 2015;40(8):755-761. doi:10.1139/apnm-2014-0530

12. Kim IY, Deutz NEP, Wolfe RR. Update on maximal anabolic response to dietary protein. *Clin Nutr.* 2018;37(2):411-418. doi:10.1016/j.clnu.2017.05.029

13. Kim IY, Schutzler S, Schrader A, et al. Quantity of dietary protein intake, but not pattern of intake, affects net protein balance primarily through differences in protein synthesis in older adults. *Am J Physiol Endocrinol Metab.* 2015;308(1):E21-E28. doi:10.1152/ajpendo.00382.2014

14. Leidy HJ, Clifton PM, Astrup A, et al. The role of protein in weight loss and maintenance. *Am J Clin Nutr.* 2015;101(6):1320S-1329S. doi:10.3945/ajcn.114.084038

Other References

1. American Heart Association Nutrition Committee, Lichtenstein AH, Appel LJ, et al. Diet and lifestyle recommendations revision 2006: a scientific statement from the American Heart Association Nutrition Committee [published correction appears in Circulation. 2006 Dec 5;114(23):e629] [published correction appears in Circulation. 2006 Jul 4;114(1):e27]. *Circulation.* 2006;114(1):82-96. doi:10.1161/CIRCULATIONAHA.106.176158

2. Bellavia A, Larsson SC, Bottai M, Wolk A, Orsini N. Differences in survival associated with processed and

with nonprocessed red meat consumption. *Am J Clin Nutr*. 2014;100(3):924-929. doi:10.3945/ajcn.114.086249

3. Berger S, Raman G, Vishwanathan R, Jacques PF, Johnson EJ. Dietary cholesterol and cardiovascular disease: a systematic review and meta-analysis. *Am J Clin Nutr*. 2015;102(2):276-294. doi:10.3945/ajcn.114.100305

4. Damasceno NR, Sala-Vila A, Cofán M, et al. Mediterranean diet supplemented with nuts reduces waist circumference and shifts lipoprotein subfractions to a less atherogenic pattern in subjects at high cardiovascular risk. *Atherosclerosis*. 2013;230(2):347-353. doi:10.1016/j.atherosclerosis.2013.08.014

5. de Cabo R, Mattson MP. Effects of Intermittent Fasting on Health, Aging, and Disease [published correction appears in N Engl J Med. 2020 Jan 16;382(3):298] [published correction appears in N Engl J Med. 2020 Mar 5;382(10):978]. *N Engl J Med*. 2019;381(26):2541-2551. doi:10.1056/NEJMra1905136

6. Dong T, Guo M, Zhang P, Sun G, Chen B. The effects of low-carbohydrate diets on cardiovascular risk factors: A meta-analysis. *PLoS One*. 2020;15(1):e0225348. Published 2020 Jan 14. doi:10.1371/journal.pone.0225348

7. Estruch R, Ros E, Salas-Salvadó J, et al. Primary Prevention of Cardiovascular Disease with a Mediterranean Diet Supplemented with Extra-Virgin Olive Oil or Nuts. *N Engl J Med*. 2018;378(25):e34. doi:10.1056/NEJMoa1800389

8. Farvid MS, Ding M, Pan A, et al. Dietary linoleic acid and risk of coronary heart disease: a systematic review and meta-analysis of prospective cohort studies. *Circulation*. 2014;130(18):1568-1578.

doi:10.1161/CIRCULATIONAHA.114.010236

9. Siri-Tarino PW, Sun Q, Hu FB, Krauss RM. Meta-analysis of prospective cohort studies evaluating the association of saturated fat with cardiovascular disease. *Am J Clin Nutr*. 2010;91(3):535-546. doi:10.3945/ajcn.2009.27725

10. Hyde PN, Sapper TN, Crabtree CD, et al. Dietary carbohydrate restriction improves metabolic syndrome independent of weight loss. *JCI Insight*. 2019;4(12):e128308. Published 2019 Jun 20. doi:10.1172/jci.insight.128308

11. Johnson RK, Lichtenstein AH, Anderson CAM, et al. Low-Calorie Sweetened Beverages and Cardiometabolic Health: A Science Advisory From the American Heart Association. *Circulation*. 2018;138(9):e126-e140. doi:10.1161/CIR.0000000000000569

12. Kirkpatrick CF, Bolick JP, Kris-Etherton PM, et al. Review of current evidence and clinical recommendations on the effects of low-carbohydrate and very-low-carbohydrate (including ketogenic) diets for the management of body weight and other cardiometabolic risk factors: A scientific statement from the National Lipid Association Nutrition and Lifestyle Task Force. *J Clin Lipidol*. 2019;13(5):689-711.e1. doi:10.1016/j.jacl.2019.08.003

13. Mitrou PN, Kipnis V, Thiébaut AC, et al. Mediterranean dietary pattern and prediction of all-cause mortality in a US population: results from the NIH-AARP Diet and Health Study. *Arch Intern Med*. 2007;167(22):2461-2468. doi:10.1001/archinte.167.22.2461

14. Mozaffarian D, Micha R, Wallace S. Effects on coronary heart disease of increasing polyunsaturated fat in place of saturated fat: a systematic review and meta-analysis of randomized controlled trials. *PLoS Med*.

2010;7(3):e1000252. Published 2010 Mar 23. doi:10.1371/journal.pmed.1000252

15. Pan A, Sun Q, Bernstein AM, et al. Red meat consumption and mortality: results from 2 prospective cohort studies. *Arch Intern Med.* 2012;172(7):555-563. doi:10.1001/archinternmed.2011.2287

16. Reynolds A, Mann J, Cummings J, Winter N, Mete E, Te Morenga L. Carbohydrate quality and human health: a series of systematic reviews and meta-analyses [published correction appears in Lancet. 2019 Feb 2;393(10170):406]. *Lancet.* 2019;393(10170):434-445. doi:10.1016/S0140-6736(18)31809-9

17. Song M, Fung TT, Hu FB, et al. Association of Animal and Plant Protein Intake With All-Cause and Cause-Specific Mortality [published correction appears in JAMA Intern Med. 2016 Nov 1;176(11):1728]. *JAMA Intern Med.* 2016;176(10):1453-1463. doi:10.1001/jamainternmed.2016.4182

18. Wang DD, Li Y, Chiuve SE, et al. Association of Specific Dietary Fats With Total and Cause-Specific Mortality. *JAMA Intern Med.* 2016;176(8):1134-1145. doi:10.1001/jamainternmed.2016.2417

19. Xi B, Veeranki SP, Zhao M, Ma C, Yan Y, Mi J. Relationship of Alcohol Consumption to All-Cause, Cardiovascular, and Cancer-Related Mortality in U.S. Adults [published correction appears in J Am Coll Cardiol. 2017 Sep 19;70(12):1542]. *J Am Coll Cardiol.* 2017;70(8):913-922. doi:10.1016/j.jacc.2017.06.054

20. Zheng Y, Li Y, Satija A, et al. Association of changes in red meat consumption with total and cause specific mortality among US women and men: two prospective cohort studies. *BMJ.* 2019;365:l2110. Published 2019 Jun 12. doi:10.1136/bmj.l2110

21. Zhong VW, Van Horn L, Greenland P, et al.

Associations of Processed Meat, Unprocessed Red Meat, Poultry, or Fish Intake With Incident Cardiovascular Disease and All-Cause Mortality. *JAMA Intern Med.* 2020;180(4):503-512. doi:10.1001/jamainternmed.2019.6969

Chap 7. Putting it all together: Progress, Adjustment, and Steady State Best

Do not set targets, just direction

Most people who start an exercise and diet plan will usually do the following:

1. They will come up with a specific weight or size or number or look they would like to get to. Usually, it's a fairly aggressive target.
2. They will pick a very restrictive diet plan and aggressive exercise plan that involves a lot of changes all at once.

Most people will make decent progress towards their target in a few months, but not actually get there. Rather than persisting, they will feel frustration and failure, and eventually give up and stop doing anything.

Some people will stick with their regimen long enough to hit the target. They will feel a sense of great accomplishment, which deserves a reward. The reward usually means loosening up on their diet and exercise regimen, and then soon they start losing all the progress they made.

Setting aggressive targets sets us up for failure. Making too many changes at once makes us feel deprived and does not allow our bodies to fully adjust to and get comfortable with the changes we make. If the changes do not become easier, it becomes impossible to continue them for the rest of your life. When you make a change, you need to know that you can stick to it most of the time for the rest of your life.

Do not set targets.
Rather than set targets, I recommend you only decide which direction you would like to make progress in. It does not matter how slowly you make progress, as long as you make some. In fact, the slower, the better. Once you hit a plateau, you make another adjustment to keep going only if you think the adjustment is something you can still stick to lifelong.

If it were possible, everyone would choose the following program: gain muscle, lose fat, and do it as fast as possible. Unfortunately, no matter what other diet programs claim (mainly to make money), this is not really possible based on how fat and muscle work.

Essentially, without setting a specific target, you need to decide on one of the following "directions of change"
1. I want more muscle without putting on too much extra fat
2. I want to lose fat, while hopefully maintaining my muscle
3. I am happy and healthy where I am, and I need to stay here

In summary,
Impatience for results is our worst enemy.
"It's not the destination, it's the journey."

Measuring yourself
Unlike many "crash" or "speed" programs, this program is going to stress the importance of making a small amount of progress over a long period of time as the only true way to achieve long term lifelong success. You must have an exercise journal or worksheet to measure your progress over time. It can be written or electronic, but you need to enter data into it regularly so you can see changes in your muscle or fat and

continue to make small adjustments in your diet and exercise routine.

The road to getting healthier is all about your ability to micro-measure and make micro-adjustments.

You will need to be consistent about recording the following:

1. Your workout progress. In Chapter 4, I provided an example of an excel worksheet that I use to keep track of every workout. For resistance workouts, you need to keep track of your strength. For aerobic workouts, you need to keep track of your aerobic ability (either calories burned, distance travelled, speed, etc.) If you are trying to lose fat or keep it down, you will also need to track your total daily activity with a fitness tracker.

2. Your weight. Weigh yourself regularly (once a day or every other day). Preferably just after you have had a bowel movement and before you have eaten anything. This gives you a sense of your usual variation depending on your hydration, salt intake, and the amount of food in your belly. Most people vary by 1-3 pounds, but some people can vary by more. It is important to realize that being 2 lbs. more than you were yesterday does not necessarily mean you have gained extra muscle or fat. However, if your highest and lowest weights are about 2 lbs. more than they were a few months ago, then you probably have gained some extra muscle (hopefully) or fat. Weighing yourself at least every other day is one of the most important things you can do to maintain your weight. Based on my experience with patients trying to lose weight, almost all of them regained it when they were not checking their weight. Sometimes this was unintentional because they hadn't made it a habit, and sometimes it was intentional because they did not want

to know the truth.   The literature supports the importance of regularly weighing yourself as well. (Thomas)

3. Measure your waist size occasionally. Use a cloth tape measure wrapped around your midsection just above your hip bone (or about halfway between the lowest portion of your ribs and your hip bone) after you breathe out. A less precise but more convenient way to stay aware of your waist size is to keep an eye on how your best fitting pants fit and if the hole you use on your most used belt changes. However, if you have a belly that sticks up over your pants, you need to use the tape measure and the method above.

4. Look at yourself in the mirror and "guesstimate "your total body fat percentage and muscle growth. You can get a reasonable sense of whether you are gaining or losing muscle and fat just based on how you look. Make sure to look at your back and legs and your posture. Men who only look at their front chest tend to overemphasize their chest and abdominal muscles over the larger and more important back and leg muscles. If you truly want to be scientific, you can use body calipers to estimate your total body fat.   I will explain this in more detail next.   However, I am not sure it is important to be that precise. Most people can have a pretty good sense just by looking in the mirror on whether they see more or less muscle around their chest, legs, and arms, and whether they see more or less fat around their waist and belly.

"Guesstimating" your total body fat percentage

When I talked about fat, I stressed that the most important risk for disease was having a lot of abdominal fat leading to a large waist circumference. When it comes to preventing disease, this is clearly true, and if you consider yourself to have a very large waist in the obese range (for example a waist size getting close to or greater than 40 inches), trying to decrease your overall waist size over time will be your main priority.

However, if your waist size is already relatively healthy (i.e., 35 inches or less), it is probably okay to let your total body fat percentage influence your plan. Trying to keep your overall body fat down is more about looking good than being healthier, but if you are doing all this work to be healthier anyway, it cannot hurt to look good as well. And it certainly can be motivating. However, once again, you need to be realistic and choose a look that is truly sustainable and achievable on a daily basis.

Following is a chart from the American College of Sports Medicine. I have rounded the numbers from the actual chart so it is less confusing. If you are at the border of a fitness level and it is really important for you to know exactly what level you are at (it should not be), then you can easily find the precise numbers on the internet. Remember though, it is very unlikely that you will be able to measure your total body fat with any kind of precision any way.

As you look at the chart to follow, it is important to recognize a few important things:

1. The fitness levels aren't really scientifically proven to affect long term health or longevity. Mainly they are just based on measuring a bunch of people they consider to have excellent fitness, good fitness, average fitness, etc. and telling you what body fat numbers they found. In addition, there is genetic and racial variation. Some racial groups may remain healthy at below average body fat level, while other racial groups may have an increased risk of disease in the average level.

2. As you age, you are allowed to have a lot more body fat.

So, a 50 year old with 16% body fat (excellent) actually gets to "outbrag" a 20 year old with 10- 12% body fat.

3. Body fat ranges in the good to excellent category are somewhat sustainable for people who are disciplined and devoted to their exercise and diet routine. Body fat ranges that are lower than numbers in the excellent range are usually not sustainable, and only achieved for short amounts of time for a competition, photo shoots, or other specific reasons to look good for a short period of time.

MEN	AGE				
Fitness Level	20's	30's	40's	50's	60 +
Excellent	7-9	11-14	14-16	15-18	15-18
Good	9-14	14-17	16-20	18-21	18-22
Average	14-17	17-20	20-22	21-24	22-25
Below Average	17-22	20-24	22-26	24-27	25-28
Poor	>22	>24	>26	>27	

WOMEN	AGE				
Fitness Level	20's	30's	40's	50's	60 +
Excellent	14-17	15-18	18-21	22-25	21-25
Good	17-21	18-22	21-25	25-28	25-29
Average	21-24	22-25	25-28	28-32	29-32
Below Average	24-28	25-29	28-32	32-35	32-36
Poor	>28	>29	>32	>35	>36

Measuring your body fat percentage is notoriously difficult. The only truly accurate measurements involve calculating your total body density using water submersion or air displacement in a special laboratory. Using "body fat" scales that use electrical impedance to calculate body fat are not accurate.

The second most accurate method without a body density laboratory is using body calipers to measure the fat thickness in different parts of your body. Usually, you will use the calipers to pinch and measure the fat under skin on your chest, abdomen, and thigh. Most calipers will come with detailed instructions and a chart. Doing a seven site measurement is usually a bit more accurate. Although the instructions on how to use the calipers appears detailed, picking the correct part of the body and knowing how to pinch the skin accurately is somewhat of an art. It's not clear that most of us can do it accurately or reliably.

Ultimately, if you have a normal waist size that does not seem to increase or decrease that much even when you gain or lose some weight, the most convenient thing to do is to just "guesstimate" your range of total body fat by looking in the mirror. In this range, it's all about how you look anyway. And if you are in the overweight or obese range, trying to decrease your waist size will ultimately be a better indicator of progress and health than calculating body fat percentage.

Below are some general guidelines on how to "guesstimate" your body fat, although there is a lot of variations between individuals, and the amount of muscle you have will clearly influence how you look as well. Someone who is a bit flabby without any muscle may overestimate their body fat simply because they don't have any muscle to give their body form and definition. Also, some people have large obvious veins, and others do not, no matter what their body fat.

<8%: muscles are defined and you can see the different muscle borders clearly (like your individual oblique muscles), skin look very thin, large veins on your upper arms, legs, and abs. As mentioned before, this is a temporary look.

10%: muscles are still quite well defined. Although you cannot see the individual oblique muscles (side abdominal muscles) as sharply, this is still a very athletic "model" look. You can see all the muscles in the abdominal six pack relatively well. There are visible veins on the upper arms and legs. Some men in their 20's may be able to sustain this.

15%: muscles are not as well defined, but you can still see the upper abdominal muscles, but maybe not the lower abdominal muscles. Usually, a slim waist and well proportioned. Still looks very lean, and athletic in clothes. The veins in the upper arms are harder to see.

20%: Muscles are not as well defined, but you can still see them. The 6 pack is almost gone but you can make it out, and there is a paunch and more obvious "love handles" than at 15%. You may make out muscles in the arms that shadow but may not see any veins in the upper arms.

25%: Muscles are not separated and blend into each other. There are no veins, and the waist is as wide as the chest.

30% and above: In this range the waist starts to be greater than 40 inches, and is probably wider than the chest and hips, and probably hanging over the beltline.

Choosing your direction

The direction you choose will be based on where you are now. As I said before, you have to choose one of three "directions of change"

1. I want to lose fat, while hopefully maintaining my muscle
2. I want more muscle without putting on too much extra fat
3. I am happy and healthy where I am, and I need to stay here

Most men will fall into one of the categories below.

You: Large waist, and a high body fat percentage in the below average or poor category.
Your direction:
    1. Lose fat, and maintain your muscle

If you consider yourself overweight, or obese, your main focus should be on losing fat and getting your waist size down. You will need to take in fewer calories than you use, forcing your body to "eat itself" by extracting energy from the fat you already have. Your weight training will make your muscle more effective and stronger, while burning calories. You may possibly gain a small amount of muscle mass in the beginning. However, you should not eat enough to gain very much. The good news is that many men who are overweight start out with a decent amount of muscle because they have been moving around the extra weight for so long. On the other hand, you do not want to cut your calories too much. If you do, you will feel deprived and hungry and tired. You will not have enough energy to repair your muscle after exercise and you may get weaker.

You: Normal waist, body fat in the average/good category. Low muscle, "flabby" "weak"
Your direction:
    2. Gain muscle, try to minimize fat gain.

You: Normal waist, body fat in the average/good/excellent category, Medium muscle in your legs and arms, with a somewhat strong, athletic look. (Mesomorph)
Your direction:
    1.2. or 3. You can choose any of the three directions above and probably still be okay.

A lot is going to depend on your personal preference of what makes you feel like your best self. You may be close or already at your desired long term "steady state". Or you may be okay with being a little weaker but looking a little leaner, especially if you have any joints that hurt more with weight. Or you may want to be stronger and bigger.

You: Skinny waist, skinny legs and arms, body fat in the good/excellent range. Very little muscle and very little fat, stereotypical "beanpole", "hard gainer", (ectomorph)
Your direction:
    2. Gain muscle, and you will probably need to take in a lot of extra calories to do so.

The Plan for Each Direction

Lose fat, maintain muscle
You: Large waist, and a high body fat percentage in the below average/poor category.
Your direction:
Lose fat, and maintain your muscle
Your main focus should be on losing fat and getting your waist size down.

Here are the steps, which involves making adjustments every two weeks.

1. Measure your baseline weight, waist size, and "guesstimate" your muscle and fat

2. Start using a calorie counting app. DO NOT make too many changes to your diet yet and do not lower your calories just yet, because increasing your exercise will increase your metabolism and hunger. If you are eager to make a change to your diet, try not to eat any food that has more than 10 grams (2 ½ teaspoons) of sugar in it. Also start to look for foods with more protein. Right now your main focus is to improve your awareness about the amount of protein, fat, carbs, and total calories you eat on a regular day.

3. Start your exercise program: weights and aerobic

4. Take a protein shake with 40+ grams of protein on the day of your workout, the next day, and any day you feel sore.

5. Weigh yourself every day or at least every other day. Measure your waist once a week.

6. WAIT. If you were exercising regularly before this, wait at least two weeks before making any changes to your diet. If you were not exercising regularly before this, wait

at least four weeks. That is right, do not make drastic changes to your diet for four weeks.

7. At 2 WEEKS (or 4 weeks if you were not exercising before) assess your direction and how you feel about your new routine. Have you lost a little weight? Is your waist measurement any smaller? Do you look like you have less fat? Are you feeling comfortable in your new routine and feel like you could continue it for another five years if you had to? Or are you struggling with hunger or cravings?

   a. Your waist size or weight is lower, you have lost some fat, and you are comfortable: Keep going another two weeks. Your routine is working, so do not change it.

   b. Your waist size or weight is lower, you have lost some fat, but you are struggling with hunger and cravings. Look for strategies to help with hunger and cravings. Try to increase the percentage of protein in your diet as much as possible, and make sure you are drinking enough water. Use protein shakes or protein snacks (nuts, Greek yogurt, etc.) to satisfy any hunger between meals. SUBSTITUTE rather than eliminate. Try to replace sugar and high glycemic carbs with lower glycemic carbs, salads, and fruits. Make the changes and continue for another two weeks

   c. You have not lost weight, your waist size is the same, and you are comfortable. Look at your food log and think about some ways you can reduce your total daily calories by 200-300 calories a day. Is there a routine snack or high calorie drink that you should get rid of? Are you eating before you go to bed? Do not try to reduce much more than 200-300 calories a day unless you have actually gained weight. SUBSTITUTE rather than eliminate. Try to replace sugar and high glycemic carbs with proteins, lower glycemic carbs, salads, and fruits. Make the changes and continue another two weeks

d. You have not lost weight, your waist size is the same, and you are struggling with hunger and cravings. This is the most frustrating situation to be in. It means your body is concerned about your losing weight, and trying to make it as hard as possible. Look closely at what you are doing and what small adjustments you can make to help with both. Are your maintaining a minimum level of activity every day (i.e., your 10,000 steps or more). Can you increase the intensity of your workouts? Try to increase the amount of protein in your diet as much as possible, and make sure you are drinking enough water. Use protein shakes or protein snacks (nuts, Greek yogurt, etc.) to lessen any hunger between meals. Once again, SUBSTITUTE rather than eliminate. Try to replace sugar and high glycemic carbs with proteins, lower glycemic carbs, salads, and fruits. Make the changes and continue another two weeks. Make the changes and continue for another two weeks.

8. Every two weeks go back to step 7 for your next set of adjustments. Continue until you one day reach a slimmer waist (at least less than 40 inches) and you feel you are in the average/good body fat percentage category. If you are significantly overweight or obese, this program is not specifically designed to help you lose an extremely large amount of fat and weight quickly. The problem is that there really is no specific diet and

exercise program that has been shown to successfully help you lose a large amount of weight quickly and then keep it off for a long period of time. Like many weight loss programs, you should be able to lose anywhere from 5 to 20% of your starting weight initially. However, unlike faster programs, the hope is that adopting changes and losing weight slowly will allow your body to reset its weight "setpoint" rather than your metabolism fighting against you. Hopefully this will help you stay committed and keep making adjustments over a long period of time. This will help you with continued fat loss and the ability to maintain a lower weight and body fat percentage for many years.

Gain muscle, minimize fat gain

You: Normal waist, body fat in the average/good category. Low muscle, "flabby" "weak"

Your direction:

Gain muscle, try to minimize fat gain.

You will need to focus on increasing your muscle, but you want to keep a close eye on not overeating and gaining fat as well. Here are the steps

1. Measure your baseline weight, waist size, and "guesstimate" your muscle and fat

2. Start using a calorie counting app. Do not make too many changes to your diet yet and do not adjust or increase your calories just yet. If you are eager to make a change to your diet, try to decrease your sugar and start to look for foods with more protein. Right now your main focus is to improve your awareness about the amount of protein, fat, carbs, and total calories you eat on a regular day.

3. Start your exercise program: weights and aerobic. You have to push yourself in your weight workouts, but keep good form and do not injure yourself.

4. Take a protein shake with 40+ grams of protein on the day of your workout, the next day, and any day you feel sore. If you are not too worried about gaining a little fat, take a protein shake every day if you want.

5. Weigh yourself every day or at least every other day. Measure your waist once a week.

6. WAIT. If you were exercising regularly before this, wait at least two weeks before making any changes to your diet. If you were not exercising regularly before this, wait at least four weeks

7. At 2 WEEKS (or 4 weeks if you were not exercising before) assess your direction and how you feel about your new routine. Have you gained muscle? Has your

strength increased? Can you lift your weights a few more times per rep than you did before? Or can you lift a few more pounds than you did a few weeks ago? Is your waist the same size? Does the amount of fat you have on your body look acceptable? Are you feeling comfortable in your new routine and feel like you could continue it for another five years if you had to?

a. You have gained strength and possibly some muscle, do not look fatter, and you are comfortable: Great job! Keep going another two weeks.

b. You have gained strength and muscle, but also looking a little fatter or "more doughy" than you would like, or your waist size is a bit more. Or you have gained some weight and are not sure how much is muscle and how much is fat. Try to maximize the percentage of calories you get with protein. Decrease your sugar as much as you can without having cravings, and still keep counting your calories and protein percentage. Make the changes and continue for another two weeks

c. You have not gained strength or muscle, and otherwise feel the same. In the beginning, if you are performing your workouts correctly, you should notice increases in strength even without gaining weight or actual muscle mass. However, after the first few months, you will need to increase your muscle mass to increase your strength. And to do this, you will need to increase your protein calories. Make sure you are getting enough protein for the medium performance range (75% of your body weight in pounds x grams protein per day). If you are already doing this, you can increase your total number of calories per day by 200-400 calories per day at most.

d. You have not gained much muscle and strength, and only feel fatter. This can only be explained by your workouts making you hungrier and you eating more, but not making good food choices with your diet. Once again, try to maximize protein, minimize sugar, and keep counting your calories and your protein/carb/fat percentage. Do not try to reduce your total calories unless you have actually gained weight. Also make sure you are really pushing yourself with your workouts. Muscle growth requires muscle damage. Make the changes and continue another two weeks

8. Every two weeks go back to step 7 for your next set of adjustments. Your goal is to always notice some progress in your strength every month for most of your free weight exercises. Continue until you reach your "steady state best", where you feel reasonably strong and athletic for your age.

Gain, gain, gain muscle

You: Skinny waist, skinny legs and arms, body fat in the good/excellent range. Very little muscle and very little fat, stereotypical "beanpole", "hard gainer", (ectomorph)

Your direction:

Gain muscle, and you will probably need to take in a lot of extra calories to do so.

If you are the stereotypical "beanpole" you can focus on increasing muscle without worrying too much about gaining fat as well. You may genetically have a high baseline metabolism, so you will need to increase your calories by a lot to promote muscle growth.

Here are the steps

1. Measure your baseline weight, waist size, and "guesstimate" your muscle and fat.

2. Start using a calorie counting app. Your main focus is to improve your awareness about the amount of protein, fat, carbs, and total calories you eat on a regular day. Make sure you are getting enough protein for the medium performance range (75% of your body weight in pounds x grams protein per day). Try to eat three meals a day minimum. For you, it is okay to have high protein snacks.

3. Start your exercise program: weights and aerobic. When you have an extra day, choose weights over aerobic.

4. Take a protein shake with 40+ grams of protein on the day of your workout, the next day, and any day you feel sore. If possible, take one every day.

5. Weigh yourself every day or at least every other day. Measure your waist once a week.

6. WAIT. If you were exercising regularly before this, wait at least two weeks before making any changes to your diet. If you were not exercising regularly before this, wait

at least four weeks

7. At 2 WEEKS (or 4 weeks if you were not exercising before) assess your direction and how you feel about your new routine. Have you gained muscle? Has your strength increased? Can you lift your weights a few more times per rep than you did before? Or can you lift a few more pounds than you did a few weeks ago? Is your waist the same size? Does the amount of fat you have on your body look acceptable? Are you feeling comfortable in your new routine and feel like you could continue it for another five years if you had to?

   a. You have gained strength and possibly some muscle, do not look fatter, and you are comfortable: Great job! Keep going another two weeks.

   b. You have not gained strength or muscle, and otherwise feel the same. In the beginning, if you are performing your workouts correctly, you should notice increases in strength even without gaining weight or actual muscle mass. However, after the first few months, you will need to increase your muscle mass to increase your strength. And to do this, you will need to increase your protein calories. Make sure you are getting enough protein for the medium performance range (75% of your body weight in pounds x grams protein per day). If you are already doing this, you can increase your total number of calories per day by 300-500 calories per day.

   c. You have gained strength and muscle, but also looking a little fatter or "more doughy" than you would like. Try to maximize the percentage of calories you get with protein. Decrease your sugar as much as you can without having cravings, and still keep counting your calories and protein percentage. Make the changes and continue for another two weeks

    d. You have not gained much muscle and only feel fatter. This can only be explained by your workouts making you hungrier, but not making good food choices with your diet. Once again, try to maximize protein, minimize sugar, and keep counting your calories and your protein/carb/fat percentage. Also make sure you are really pushing yourself with your workouts. Muscle growth requires muscle damage. Make the changes and continue another two weeks

8. Every two weeks go back to step 7 for your next set of adjustments. Your goal is to always notice some progress in your strength every month for most of your free weight exercises. Continue until you reach your "steady state best", where you feel reasonably strong and athletic for your age.

Hunger and Muscle Growth

When you are struggling with hunger and cravings but not losing fat, it is tempting to reduce calories drastically to get better fat loss, but this will only make the hunger worse. It is not sustainable. Losing more than 1lb every week is too much if you are continuously feeling hungry doing it. It is better to focus on finding ways to let your hunger become manageable before pushing yourself further.

Muscle growth requires muscle damage, which means you have to push yourself with every workout. However, for most people, the rate of muscle growth is very slow and capped no matter how much you work out and no matter how much you eat. So, although overdoing both working out and eating excessively will help bodybuilders and actors get in shape for their roles, it is not a realistic long-term plan for most of us. Overeating to build muscle will also increase your fat, and get you used to eating big meals. This makes it harder to lose the fat you just gained. So even if you are not gaining muscle as fast as you would like, it is better to eat just enough extra protein to help you gain some muscle without putting on extra fat.

The key to long term success is making very small adjustments over many months until you get to your "steady state best."

Measure your cardiovascular fitness

Along with improvements in your body composition, you should be able to see improvements in your aerobic workouts. With your activities, make sure to measure your time and distance if possible. With time you should be able to go further and faster.

Your "steady state best". Time to maintain

At a certain point you have to decide on the best version of yourself that is sustainable. Much of your ability to put on muscle or to lower your waist fat will be genetically limited. Even though you could theoretically push through these limits, it usually is not sustainable unless you devote your life to it. Hopefully you have better ways to live your life. Work as hard as you can to gain muscle and lose your waist fat, but at a certain point you have to decide what you can realistically maintain. **Sustainability is the key concept.** For most men, keeping your body fat in the average or good range is both healthy and sustainable. For those men who started with a very large waist, it may be extremely hard to get to a more normal size waist without feeling perpetually hungry. In this case the goal is to get to as low a waist size as possible without feeling it is too hard. In terms of muscle, at a certain point you may feel that you are maxed out at the amount of muscle you have gained. At this point if you continue the same workout you may not see any increases in strength. That is okay, as long as you don't see a decrease in strength. You may be tempted to add additional workouts to increase your muscle size, which is fine. However, be aware that you may lose that additional muscle and strength once you stop doing the additional workouts.

Once you have reached your steady state, you can't just relax. You need to continue the same diet and workout you have been doing until this point. The only difference is that you are not adjusting to increase your strength or lower your fat. You are working to just stay at your steady state. In many ways this is often the hardest phase to maintain motivation because you are no longer seeing the positive effects of your work. However, you have to remind yourself that without maintaining your routine, you will start to lose the progress you made. Meaning you may regain some fat and lose some muscle.

You will still have to make good food choices and commit to finding the time to exercise. You will always have to make some micro adjustments. And you will still have to commit to pushing yourself as hard as possible with each workout. But hopefully after several months, you should feel that you can make the appropriate food choices and follow the basic workout schedule for the rest of your life. If you are happy with your strength and muscle mass, you probably do not have to take protein shakes and extra protein (unless you are a beanpole hard gainer). You can even drop down to minimum protein need, which is about 50% of your body weight in pounds x grams of protein per day. Or you may find you feel better still taking protein shakes on the days of your weight workouts. If you notice yourself holding a bit more fat than usual, you will have to be stricter about following your diet guidelines. At this stage, you should know enough about your own body and how it responds to your routine, and make the needed adjustments continually.

Overall, you should feel great for your age, or any age. You should be able to be active throughout the day, and more capable of moving and lifting than you were before. You should have more strength to avoid injury, more stamina for activity, and more reserve to get through illnesses. You should feel more optimistic about your ability to feel healthy and capable even as you grow older. And hopefully that is more than enough motivation to keep you going.

Calorie Counting App Predictions: Ignore Them

I want to add a final note for those of you who do a very thorough job of counting the calories you eat every day AND the calories you burn every day. Keeping track of both is absolutely a great thing to do, but DO NOT USE the predictions many of the calorie counting apps will give you about your weight. These predictions are made using very simple generic formulas where they take the amount of calories you eat and subtract some generic amount of basal metabolism along with the calories you burned, and then predict how much weight you will gain or lose. First of all, the calories you enter are just very rough estimates, and not truly accurate measurements of what you are eating and burning. Second, everyone has a different basal metabolism. And lastly, there are hundreds of factors that will affect your metabolism and how you gain or lose weight. So ultimately, you must measure your actual results, and base your predictions on what you learn about yourself. You do have to measure your progress with exercise and activity, but you should not measure it using calories. Perhaps in the near future, the apps will incorporate some type of machine learning or improved algorithms to achieve more accurate predictions, but right now you are going to have to do that yourself.

Summary

1. **Sustainability** and **lifelong** is the key concept. Slow small changes that you can imagine practicing over a lifetime will be more successful in the long run than drastic ones.
2. Do not set goals, only the direction you want to head towards. You have a choice of three directions:
   a. I want more muscle without putting on too much extra fat
   b. I want to lose fat, while hopefully maintaining my muscle
   c. I am happy and healthy where I am, and I need to stay here
3. You need to continually make small "micro" adjustments to your diet and exercise to see progress in the direction you want. You have to be fully aware of how you are exercising and how you are eating in order to measure progress or lack of progress. If you cannot measure, you

cannot adjust. You must measure regularly for the rest of your life.

4. Measuring your exercise involves measuring the weight you can lift, and the improvements in your aerobic workouts.
5. Measuring your diet involves calorie counting, minimizing sugar, and maximizing protein.
6. Measuring yourself involves measuring your weight, your waist size, and "guesstimating" your body fat percentage. At minimum, you should weigh yourself several times a week for the rest of your life.

References

1. Anderson JW, Konz EC, Frederich RC, Wood CL. Long-term weight-loss maintenance: a meta-analysis of US studies. *Am J Clin Nutr.* 2001;74(5):579-584. doi:10.1093/ajcn/74.5.579
2. Asbjørnsen RA, Smedsrød ML, Solberg Nes L, et al. Persuasive System Design Principles and Behavior Change Techniques to Stimulate Motivation and Adherence in Electronic Health Interventions to Support Weight Loss Maintenance: Scoping Review. *J Med Internet Res.* 2019;21(6):e14265. Published 2019 Jun 21. doi:10.2196/14265
3. Camps SG, Verhoef SP, Westerterp KR. Weight loss, weight maintenance, and adaptive thermogenesis [published correction appears in Am J Clin Nutr. 2014 Nov;100(5):1405]. *Am J Clin Nutr.* 2013;97(5):990-994. doi:10.3945/ajcn.112.050310
4. Ebbeling CB, Feldman HA, Klein GL, et al. Effects of a low carbohydrate diet on energy expenditure during weight loss maintenance: randomized trial [published correction appears in BMJ. 2020 Nov 3;371:m4264].

BMJ. 2018;363:k4583. Published 2018 Nov 14. doi:10.1136/bmj.k4583

5. Elfhag K, Rössner S. Who succeeds in maintaining weight loss? A conceptual review of factors associated with weight loss maintenance and weight regain. *Obes Rev.* 2005;6(1):67-85. doi:10.1111/j.1467-789X.2005.00170.x

6. Hall KD, Kahan S. Maintenance of Lost Weight and Long-Term Management of Obesity. *Med Clin North Am.* 2018;102(1):183-197. doi:10.1016/j.mcna.2017.08.012

7. Hintze LJ, Mahmoodianfard S, Auguste CB, Doucet É. Weight Loss and Appetite Control in Women. *Curr Obes Rep.* 2017;6(3):334-351. doi:10.1007/s13679-017-0273-8

8. Phillips SM. A brief review of higher dietary protein diets in weight loss: a focus on athletes. *Sports Med.* 2014;44 Suppl 2(Suppl 2):S149-S153. doi:10.1007/s40279-014-0254-y

9. Rosenbaum M, Heaner M, Goldsmith RL, et al. Resistance Training Reduces Skeletal Muscle Work Efficiency in Weight-Reduced and Non-Weight-Reduced Subjects. *Obesity (Silver Spring).* 2018;26(10):1576-1583. doi:10.1002/oby.22274

10. Thomas JG, Bond DS, Phelan S, Hill JO, Wing RR. Weight-loss maintenance for 10 years in the National Weight Control Registry. *Am J Prev Med.* 2014;46(1):17-23. doi:10.1016/j.amepre.2013.08.019

11. Wall BT, Morton JP, van Loon LJ. Strategies to maintain skeletal muscle mass in the injured athlete: nutritional considerations and exercise mimetics. *Eur J Sport Sci.* 2015;15(1):53-62. doi:10.1080/17461391.2014.936326

12. Wing RR, Phelan S. Long-term weight loss

maintenance. *Am J Clin Nutr.* 2005;82(1 Suppl):222S-225S. doi:10.1093/ajcn/82.1.222S

13. Westerterp-Plantenga MS, Lemmens SG, Westerterp KR. Dietary protein - its role in satiety, energetics, weight loss and health. *Br J Nutr.* 2012;108 Suppl 2:S105-S112. doi:10.1017/S0007114512002589

14. Yannakoulia M, Poulimeneas D, Mamalaki E, Anastasiou CA. Dietary modifications for weight loss and weight loss maintenance. *Metabolism.* 2019;92:153-162. doi:10.1016/j.metabol.2019.01.001

Chap 8. How to Stay Motivated Lifelong

I believe this program is completely sustainable for years and decades. However, maintaining motivation for a long time is hard, especially if you are impatient and want to see faster improvements. Continuing a routine like this lifelong can be difficult, which is why your mindset is important.

This is the part where trainers will tell you that you have "to give it 110%". "No pain, no gain." "Extreme and absolute focus is the key to success." "Good is not enough when better is possible."

Although this kind of mindset makes sense for athletes, bodybuilders, and superhero actors, it is not a sustainable mindset for most of us. The "always give it 100%" approach, leads to all or nothing thinking. Some days we just can't give it 110%. Some days, we can give only 50%, and that's okay.

So my slogans for mindset include the following:
"Some progress is better than no progress."
"Give it whatever you can, whenever you can."
"Half ass is better than no ass."
Sorry to include the last one, which is somewhat crude, but unfortunately the most memorable.

Avoid all or nothing thinking

As I mentioned before, when we are overly rigid about following a diet, if we ultimately break the "rules", we rightfully conclude that it will be impossible to follow these rules lifelong. This conclusion, along with the shame of giving in, usually convinces us to abandon the entire diet completely. Try to avoid this "all or nothing" thinking. Your goal is to eat healthy most of the time, but not all of the time. That is the only way most of us can maintain a truly healthy diet for the next 10, 20, or 50 years.

When you work out, sometimes you just don't have enough energy or motivation to lift your heaviest weights or run your fastest run. That's okay. Lift lighter, run slower. You will at least maintain your fitness, and still might make some small gains.

Similarly, there may be legitimate reasons you may not be able to exercise for a few weeks, or even a few months. Life happens. Have faith that when you restart your body has both muscle memory and cardiovascular fitness memory, so that you will regain your original strength and fitness much sooner than you think.

Just start. Don't worry about the finish.

Sometimes you may not have enough time, energy, or motivation to do a workout. You may not have an hour to lift weights. Or you feel too tired to run 3 miles. Tell yourself you will just do a mini workout. Maybe you just spend 15 minutes doing leg exercises. Maybe you tell yourself you will run just one mile. Many times, if you still have additional time, you will find that once you start it is not too hard to keep going. Maybe you add another 15 minutes for another set of weights. Or maybe you decide you feel energetic enough to run a second mile. Or maybe you don't that day. That's okay. In other words, if the task ahead seems too big, you are less likely to start it. But if you make the task small, you are more likely to start it. And once you start, you sometimes find you have the momentum to take on more.

Focus on what you did, not what you didn't

I've had several dogs throughout my life, and one of the most memorable pieces of advice a dog trainer once gave was, "You cannot tell a dog to not do something. If you don't want your dog doing something, you have to tell it what to do instead." "If you don't want your dog to jump, reward her for sitting. If you don't want it to bark, reward him for being quiet. If you don't want her to beg at the dinner table, teach her to down-stay far away."

Similarly, celebrate what you do right. Do not obsess about what you didn't do or didn't do right. If you didn't exercise for three weeks, congratulate yourself for starting up again. If you drank too much alcohol and ate too much cake at a party last night, make a commitment to get out your calorie counting app again. Of course, when I say celebrate, I mean congratulate yourself on your dedication to good health. Don't celebrate with more alcohol and cake.

Are you loving this yet?

Enjoying exercise, enjoying making good food choices, and enjoying how you feel is the hardest part of any program. However, it is the single most important part of motivation if you want to keep going.

When something requires effort, people do not always do what they know is good for them. But they usually do what they enjoy and love. If you cannot get to the point where you somewhat enjoy your workouts, then even three hours a week is going to seem like torture. And that is going to be very hard to keep up for the rest of your life.

The other reason you need to enjoy your good health is because, when it comes to food, you are frequently depriving yourself of foods you know taste good. Many people love the thought and taste of food. They look forward to eating certain foods hours or even days before they eat them. Some people look forward to a dinner with friends because they look forward to the friendship, while others actually look forward to the dinner itself. If you are one of those people who "loves" food, then even putting mild restrictions on your food is going to be very difficult. You will feel constantly "deprived."

You cannot go through life feeling constantly deprived. If you can't let go of your love of food, you must substitute it with something healthy you love more. You have to use your health and fitness to experience life in ways that you love. When my patients tell me how excited they are about hiking, horseback riding, running 5K races, travelling, or walking with their kids through Disneyland, they also tell me that the sacrifices around food are worth it. It makes choosing the right foods and avoiding the unhealthy ones easier when they have something else to look forward to.

If you cannot let go of your love of food, you will also need to really look at your relationship with food. Addressing how to do this is beyond the scope of this book, and you will need to look at other books, classes, support groups, or forms of therapy. In general, if food makes you feel loved, or brings you joy, or soothes your emotions, then you will have to find a healthier way to experience those same feelings. You cannot go through life feeling unloved or joyless.

Chap 9. Your inner self.

Emotional and mental health is just as important as your physical health. The two are synergistic, since good emotional health makes it easier to commit to being physically healthy, and good physical health actually boosts positive emotions and can lower depression. (Gordon, Choi)

The many ways to improve your inner self and emotional and mental health is beyond the scope of this book. I will not try to address serious mental health issues such as depression, bipolar disorder, persistent anger, or long-standing addiction. But I will try to cram in a few tidbits that are proven to be helpful to almost all men, young or old. If you find any of these ideas interesting, I recommend exploring them further with more detailed reading, bringing them up with others, or even talking to a therapist.

The midlife crisis is real

Most men, and even women, spend the first decades of their lives trying to acquire security: a good job, a good family, a good home, and many other things that we have traditionally been taught to acquire. Those with more ambition and ego may also try to acquire power, status, wealth, and recognition. In the 1900's, most men died by the age of 50, still trying to work and survive. There was no such thing as retirement. In this day and age, we may live many decades longer, and most studies show that almost all of us will stay in the same socioeconomic status after age 40 or 50. In other words, our careers and social status do not seem to change that much after 40. We often spend the first half of our lives measuring our self-worth by what we have acquired, our careers, and our accomplishments. When we measure our worth in this way, based on "external validation", the second half of our lives can introduce low self-esteem. This is because we stop acquiring new things, our accomplishments are less, and we grow weaker and look older. Men who continue to need external validation may go through the stereotypical midlife crisis: divorce, new relationships, a new sports car, and trying to act and feel young again. Instead of accepting or grieving things they may not have done or lives they did not live, they try to redo their lives and actions. This usually does not bring them deep satisfaction or insight. Some may self-medicate their low self-esteem with addictions to alcohol, drugs, gambling, food, sex, or pornography. To be emotionally healthy, men will need to let go of self-worth that is dependent on external validation. They will need to work on their internal sense of self-worth. (Real) This is based largely on them finding meaning in their lives, as well as gratitude for all they have. They need to ask themselves what brings their inner selves meaning. (Frankel) This is also the time to literally "slow down and smell the roses." They need to appreciate the time they spend with loved ones and good friends. They need to nurture their relationships. They need to cherish time, accept their own mortality, and enjoy the experience of life. And they need to have the strength to be vulnerable and feel true to themselves.

Practice your emotional vocabulary

For some reason, naming an emotion as we are feeling it has the remarkable effect of softening the emotion.   The very act of telling yourself you are feeling angry can lessen that anger and help you control it. Which means having a better emotional vocabulary allows you to understand and control more of your emotions.

How many emotions are there?

Can you name the 6 traditional emotions most of us think of? Look below for the 6.

6 "traditional model" emotions:

Happiness
Sadness
Fear
Anger
Surprise
Disgust

A recent study based on responses to videos suggests 27 different emotions [Cowen]. Try to write down as many as possible and then check your answers against the list below. You do not have to be right or agree with the emotions they listed. What is most important is that you understand the variety of emotions and the subtle differences between them. The more you can name, the better your emotional vocabulary.

27 "Berkeley model" emotions:

Admiration
Adoration
Aesthetic Appreciation
Amusement
Anxiety
Awe
Awkwardness
Boredom
Calmness
Confusion
Craving
Disgust
Empathetic pain
Entrancement

Envy
Excitement
Fear
Horror
Interest
Joy
Nostalgia
Romance
Sadness
Satisfaction
Sexual desire
Sympathy
Triumph

Also, do you know the difference between feelings and emotions? Emotions are more primal, reactive, sudden, and intense. They come from somewhere deep within. They may or may not be understood. Feelings are like emotions that are processed, thought about, and interpreted. They are the story that is built around your emotions. You may have feelings about something even when you are not actually experiencing the emotion that influenced those feelings.

Men can express depression in many less obvious ways. When we imagine depression, we usually think of a very low energy person expressing sadness or withdrawal. However, many men who are depressed will express their depression as continual anger or frustration or bitterness. (Real) This allows them to blame external factors for their internal state.

Another common reaction to depression and underlying shame is the need for grandiosity. There are many men who must perpetually project a state of importance to others and themselves and spend all their energy maintaining that illusion. When they stop maintaining their grandiosity, they become overcome by their depression. Rather than address this, they go back to their grandiosity, which is the only way they know how to feel good about themselves.

In other words, although we traditionally think of depression as "Eyeore", sometimes depression in men can present more like "Tigger."

Practice gratitude

There are many variations of the gratitude exercise, and all of them have been proven to improve your sense of self-worth and happiness.

Every day, write or say one sentence expressing gratitude for something in your life. Or you can write three things once a week.

If possible, try to be specific about your role in it. Or explain the details of why you are grateful for something. As an example, rather than say, "I am grateful for my child", say "I am grateful for the relationship I have with my child and the time we have together. Fatherhood has changed me"

Another effective exercise is writing a letter to someone you are particularly grateful to. There are many other exercises and variations which I will not go over in detail, but try a few and see what works for you.

Journaling

Journaling is the poor person's version of therapy. It can be difficult to maintain the habit but look at the bright side: Even if you do it once a week for one hour, it's cheaper and more convenient than an hour of therapy, and has been shown to significantly improve depression, anxiety, and other negative emotions [Krapn]. There are many reasons why journaling can be therapeutic:

- It forces you to articulate your thoughts. Sometimes the thoughts you may have inside your head seem to have logic and clarity, but they are more confused or loosely formed than you realize. Writing them down forces you to find consistency, logic, and clarity in your thoughts.
- Hopefully, it pushes you to name your emotions.
- It may allow you to uncover repressed emotions, feelings, and thoughts.
- It slows and focuses your mind for self-reflection.
- It gives you the opportunity to write down your gratitude.
- It allows you to look back at what you wrote before and reflect on how time may have changed your interpretation of events.
- It allows you to define your identity. Is who you are totally in sync with who you want to be? Do others see you the way you see yourself?

Social media

Use social media wisely, and pay attention to how it is making you feel and how it is affecting your emotions. Every time you read a post, ask yourself how that made you feel or what your emotions are. If most of your feelings and emotions are more negative than positive, then social media is not helping you. Maintain your friendships and important connections through more personal methods like texting, email, and hanging out together.

Pause before posting anything argumentative, negative, or sarcastic. Even if you think it's funny. The longer the better. Not just minutes, but hours, or even a day. Sarcasm and humor do not always translate well on social media. Pause even if you think what you are saying is neutral or innocuous. Pause for humble brags about yourself. Positive messages about others are probably the only thing you do not need to pause for. (i.e., Wow, that looks amazing! Hope you have an awesome birthday! etc.)

Mental exercises help with brain health

Challenging yourself mentally is proven to preserve your brain power for longer, preventing the memory loss, lack of concentration, and dementia that can sometimes come with old age. You can make it a habit to play brain games such as crosswords, Sudoku, memory games, and word jumbles. You can find many different brain game apps. Learning a musical instrument, drawing or painting, or learning a new language can stimulate new parts of your brain and prevent dementia.

Addiction

People can become dependent and addicted to alcohol, drugs, pot, gambling, sex, porn, and many other substances or activities. But how do we know when a behavior is just casual fun or addiction? I will use alcohol as an example. When you go to a friend's party and have some alcohol, it is usually spontaneous and can add some fun to your social experience. If you have been looking forward to drinking with your friends since the morning, there is nothing wrong with that, as long as you are more excited about the upcoming social interaction rather than the act of drinking. However, if you were more excited about the drinking than the time you would spend with your friends, this becomes more concerning. If you drink a few drinks once a week, and noticeably feel like you are "missing out" if you miss a weekend, that is concerning for a habit. If you drink every day or a few times a week, no matter what the circumstance, that is clearly a habit, and probably an addiction. If you start thinking about alcohol when you are not drinking, or frequently drink alone, that is an addiction. If you drink alcohol to help when you are stressed, depressed, or in some type of negative mood, then you are dependent on alcohol to soothe you, and have an addiction. In the example above, you can replace alcohol with any type of substance or activity. In general, if you are taking a substance or engaging in an activity to help patch negative emotions and feelings, then you are at risk for addiction. If you are occasionally taking a substance or engaging in an activity to enhance an already positive state of mind, you are probably okay.

If you drink a cup of coffee every morning to wake up, is that an addiction? Possibly, but not one that ruins your life. You are dependent on it to wake up, but not necessarily to soothe a negative emotion. It is a habit, but not one that can affect your life negatively. Can you be addicted to exercise? Yes, absolutely. If it truly makes you healthier and does not affect your life negatively, then it is probably a healthy addiction. However, if you are spending less time with your significant other to exercise and it is affecting your relationship, you are doing it at the expense of your other responsibilities, or you are actually injuring yourself or putting yourself in danger, then it may be an unhealthy addiction.

You need to break dependencies and addictions, because ultimately, they control you more than you control them, and it is easier to break them earlier rather than later. You may be able to break a habit by yourself if you try. However, to break an addiction you will usually need professional help and support to address the underlying negative emotions and state of mind that fuel them.

Friendships
Numerous studies confirm that friendships are huge contributors to our happiness. As we gain a better perspective

on what is most meaningful in life, it is never too late to reconnect with old friends. And sometimes you have nothing to lose trying to create new friendships. Spend time with friends you can be yourself with.

Accept your mortality

Accepting the end of your life allows you to provide perspective to the life you are living now, and hopefully allows you to live a life without regret. It allows you to prioritize what is truly important to you, and how to best spend your time. Hopefully it allows you to live your life without fear of little things like embarrassment or rejection. Hopefully it allows you to express your emotions and vulnerability without fear. On a practical level, it is important to discuss your advanced directive with loved ones. Working on your advanced directive also forces you to really think about what is the minimum quality of life you still consider a life worth living. If you were completely paralyzed but your thoughts were intact and you could still witness the lives of the people you care about, would that be enough for you to keep living? If a stroke left you relatively independent, but erased most of your memory, would you still want to live? What is more important to you: your mental awareness or your physical ability? These are all rare unlikely scenarios and hypothetical questions, but they can help you define how you view your life. In addition, in the unfortunate situation that your loved ones must make a life or death decision for you, providing them the guidance of your true healthy voice is the best gift you can give them.

References

1. Basso JC, Shang A, Elman M, Karmouta R, Suzuki WA. Acute Exercise Improves Prefrontal Cortex but not Hippocampal Function in Healthy Adults. *J Int*

Neuropsychol   Soc.   2015;21(10):791-801. doi:10.1017/S1355617715000106

2. Choi KW, Zheutlin AB, Karlson RA, et al. Physical activity offsets genetic risk for incident depression assessed via electronic health records in a biobank cohort study. *Depress Anxiety.* 2020;37(2):106-114. doi:10.1002/da.22967

3. Choi KW, Chen CY, Stein MB, et al. Assessment of Bidirectional Relationships Between Physical Activity and Depression Among Adults: A 2-Sample Mendelian Randomization   Study.   *JAMA   Psychiatry.* 2019;76(4):399-408. doi:10.1001/jamapsychiatry.2018.4175

4. Cooney GM, Dwan K, Greig CA, et al. Exercise for depression.   Cochrane   Database   Syst   Rev. 2013;(9):CD004366.   Published   2013   Sep   12. doi:10.1002/14651858.CD004366.pub6

5. Cowen AS, Keltner D. Self-report captures 27 distinct categories of emotion bridged by continuous gradients. *Proc Natl Acad Sci U S A.* 2017;114(38):E7900-E7909. doi:10.1073/pnas.1702247114

6. Emmons RA, Stern R. Gratitude as a psychotherapeutic intervention. *J Clin Psychol.* 2013;69(8):846-855. doi:10.1002/jclp.22020

7. Gordon BR, McDowell CP, Hallgren M, Meyer JD, Lyons M, Herring MP. Association of Efficacy of Resistance Exercise Training With Depressive Symptoms: Meta-analysis and Meta-regression Analysis of Randomized Clinical Trials. *JAMA Psychiatry.* 2018;75(6):566-576. doi:10.1001/jamapsychiatry.2018.0572

8. Herring MP, Puetz TW, O'Connor PJ, Dishman RK. Effect of exercise training on depressive symptoms among patients with a chronic illness: a systematic review and meta-analysis of randomized controlled

trials. *Arch Intern Med.* 2012;172(2):101-111. doi:10.1001/archinternmed.2011.696

9. Krpan KM, Kross E, Berman MG, Deldin PJ, Askren MK, Jonides J. An everyday activity as a treatment for depression: the benefits of expressive writing for people diagnosed with major depressive disorder. *J Affect Disord.* 2013;150(3):1148-1151. doi:10.1016/j.jad.2013.05.065

10. O'Leary K, Dockray S. The effects of two novel gratitude and mindfulness interventions on well-being. *J Altern Complement Med.* 2015;21(4):243-245. doi:10.1089/acm.2014.0119

11. Schuch FB, Vancampfort D, Richards J, Rosenbaum S, Ward PB, Stubbs B. Exercise as a treatment for depression: A meta-analysis adjusting for publication bias. *J Psychiatr Res.* 2016;77:42-51. doi:10.1016/j.jpsychires.2016.02.023

12. Segal SK, Cotman CW, Cahill LF. Exercise-induced noradrenergic activation enhances memory consolidation in both normal aging and patients with amnestic mild cognitive impairment. *J Alzheimers Dis.* 2012;32(4):1011-1018. doi:10.3233/JAD-2012-121078

Books

1. Viktor E. Frankl , "Man's Search for Meaning." mult editions.
2. James Hollis. "Finding Meaning in the Second Half of Life: How to Finally, Really Grow Up." c. Mar 16, 2006
3. Gordon Livingston and Elizabeth Edwards. "Too Soon Old, Too Late Smart: Thirty True Things You Need to Know Now."Mar 4, 2008

4. Terrence Real. "I Don't Want to Talk About It: Overcoming the Secret Legacy of Male Depression." c. Mar 11, 1999

Chap 10. Your medical health

Good health depends on a good diet, regular activity, good mental health, and enough sleep. Improving these factors is the best way to improve your health and hopefully prevent or lessen diseases such as high blood pressure, heart disease, and diabetes. Avoiding substances that harm your body like cigarettes, vaping, and alcohol is equally important. Although doctors and health care workers believe in good health and improving all of the factors mentioned above, they are not with you every day to help coach and motivate you. Instead, you see them when you are sick or need to treat a disease. The healthcare system is largely built around treating disease rather than preventing it. The system is really a disease care system, rather than a health care system. Our healthcare systems can help treat cancer, chronic diseases, and injuries. But the rest of your health depends on your environment and personal choice. Most of the blue zones in the world clearly demonstrate this. Nicoya, Costa Rica spends about 15% of what America spends on healthcare per person, yet the people there are more than twice as likely to live until the age of 90 than Americans are.

Nevertheless, you still need to use the health care system intermittently to insure your optimal health. I will touch on a few things you should do to prevent disease:

Seeing your doctor

Even the healthiest man or woman should see their doctor for the following:

- Colon cancer screening once you are age 50. Colon cancer screening absolutely detects potential colon cancer in its earliest stages and can save your life. There is almost zero downside to having colon cancer screening. There is a big downside to missing a colon cancer: death.

- You should check your blood pressure every 3 years until you are age 40, and then at least once a year after age 40. Hopefully by following a regular exercise and diet program, you should not develop high blood pressure. But if you do, you should absolutely control it to prevent stroke, heart disease, and kidney disease.
- You should check your cholesterol and lipid profile (a blood test) every four or five years, or more frequently if recommended by your doctor.
- Women should have HPV tests or PAP smears regularly to prevent cervical cancer, and should start getting mammograms sometime between the ages of 40 and 50.
- If you have any left sided chest pain with activity, or pain that radiates down your left arm, you should absolutely see your doctor immediately. They will usually recommend a stress test to make sure it is not your heart. Even healthy athletes can develop heart disease if they are genetically predisposed to it.

Never be afraid to see your doctor if you feel something is "different, or not quite right". It is better to be safe, rather than let something serious go on longer than it should. If you truly do feel something is wrong, but you are not satisfied with your doctor's interpretation, do not be afraid or embarrassed to ask for a second opinion. You only have one body, and you deserve to feel comfortable about and trust the care you receive.

Screen yourself for Sleep Apnea

If you have sleep apnea, you should absolutely talk to your doctor about getting tested and treated. Sleep apnea refers to difficulty breathing correctly while asleep, and you are at risk of apnea if you have two or more of the following symptoms (STOP BANG)

S	(Snore)	Do you snore?
T	(Tired)	Do you feel tired during the day?
		Do you wake up feeling like you haven't slept?
O	(Obstruction)	Have you been told you stop breathing at night?
		Do you gasp for air or choke while sleeping?
P	(Pressure)	Do you have high blood pressure?
		Are you on a medication to control high blood pressure?

If you answer YES to two or more questions above, you should talk to your doctor about a sleep apnea test. The other factors that will also increase your risk of moderate or severe apnea include:

B: BMI high (obesity)

A: Age over 50

N: Neck circumference more than 17 inches for men, 16 inches for women

G: Gender. Being a man is a higher risk.

Treating sleep apnea helps with weight loss. When you have apnea, your tissues are not getting enough oxygen, which can cause your cells to lower your metabolism. When you fully oxygenate your tissues, you are more likely to run at your maximum metabolism, which can help you lose fat.

Aspirin

Based on many older studies, some people may have heard that taking a baby aspirin every day after age 40 can prevent a heart attack, and there is no downside. Unfortunately, aspirin does increase the risk of ulcers and bleeding, and probably should not be taken regularly unless you have risk factors for heart disease. The risk of heart disease increases with high blood pressure, diabetes, a higher risk cholesterol/lipid panel, smoking, or a strong family history. If you are not sure about your risk of a heart attack, you should discuss aspirin use with your doctor.

Even though we no longer recommend aspirin for healthy men, if you are over age 40, you can consider taking one baby aspirin (81 mg) on the day of an event such as a running event, bicycle race, a triathlon, or a Spartan race. Often you may push yourself harder than usual, and the effort along with the surge of adrenaline can slightly increase your chance of a sudden heart attack if you have some mild heart disease you are not aware of. You will have to weigh this against the chance of bleeding more if you wipe out and have an accident. Hopefully neither will be an issue and your event goes well.

Nicotine, Alcohol, Pot, and other substances.

Quitting smoking and nicotine is a no brainer. The health benefits of quitting smoking are more significant than losing fat or anything else. If you smoke, vape, chew tobacco regularly, or use nicotine regularly in any way, quitting nicotine use is more important than any other advice I provide in this book.

The same goes for drug and opioid addictions. Those addictions are life threatening and getting sober is the most important thing you can do to live longer and better. It has been said that there is no such thing as a heroin "overdose", since the word "overdose" implies that there is some correct dose. There is none. Any use is potentially life threatening.

I have already discussed alcohol. Basically, the less the better, but it does not have to be never. Keep it limited to rare social occasions.

Finally, there is no substantial research to suggest that regular pot use can shorten your life. However, most of the research related to THC and CBD is inherently flawed because of the inability in our society to design well controlled studies. Pot and THC can increase hunger, so if you are trying to keep your calories low to keep your waist size down, I would recommend that you limit pot use to nighttime only, after your last meal. Promise yourself that you will not eat anything after you use it, and its effects should be gone by the morning before breakfast.

Aging

As mentioned before, as men age, they lose testosterone and muscle mass. As both men and women age, our bodies become more efficient at living and we lower our baseline metabolism. Which means it becomes easier to gain fat when we overeat. As the brain ages, we have more problems with memory, concentration, and problem-solving ability.

Scientific studies overwhelmingly support the beneficial effects of a healthy diet and regular exercise in slowing all forms of aging. There is no controversy about it. As you age, keeping your mind challenged and learning again will slow memory loss and dementia. People in the "blue zones" not only live longer, but they also function longer. In fact, very few of them understand the word "retirement."

Your Advanced Directive.

None of us had any control of how we were born, and the

overwhelming majority of us will have no control over how we die either. However, we can have some say before it happens.

Writing your advance directive is not thinking about how you want to die; it is thinking about how you want to live. If you look at it in that light, it can be an extremely rewarding exercise in gratitude and self-reflection.

There are two components to an Advanced Directive: a living will, and a durable power of attorney.

A living will is a document that states your preference for certain medical treatments and interventions ONLY if you have terminal illness or doctors think you will be permanently unconscious. It will not be used if you are in an accident or have a short-term medical emergency that doctors think you can recover from. In that case, they are usually obligated to be aggressive in treating you. However, if you have a terminal illness, or will be permanently unconscious, the living will can be used to guide medical decisions. Each state has its own living will paperwork. Most documents will ask you about whether you would want specific interventions and treatments. These can include being on a ventilator, CPR, starting dialysis, or receiving tube feeds if you can longer eat by mouth.

The durable power of attorney names a person who can make medical decisions for you ONLY if you cannot make them for yourself (which is determined by the doctors). You need to choose a durable power of attorney you trust completely, and you need to talk to them in depth about your wishes.

As a doctor, I have seen many families struggle with the decision to let a loved one go, even when all the doctors confirm that meaningful recovery is hopeless. It is a huge responsibility for a family member to give doctors permission to let a loved die.

There are feelings of guilt and betrayal. Talking to your family members and loved ones in advance is one of the greatest gifts you can give them. Try to think about what is truly meaningful to you. What is the minimum health you need to make life worth living? For example, if you could not speak or eat on your own, but could understand what is happening around you, would you want to still keep living? If you could not remember your kids or loved ones, would you want to still keep living? If you were mentally sharp, but physically completely dependent on caretakers, would you want to still keep living? These are the kinds of scenarios and questions you should think about and discuss with loved one so that they know how to make a decision if they unfortunately need to. Knowing that they are respecting your wants and wishes about a life worth living will bring them some guidance and solace during a difficult heartbreaking time.

References

1. Arnett DK, Blumenthal RS, Albert MA, et al. 2019 ACC/AHA Guideline on the Primary Prevention of Cardiovascular Disease: A Report of the American College of Cardiology/American Heart Association Task Force on Clinical Practice Guidelines *Circulation*. 2019;140(11):e596-e646. doi:10.1161/CIR.0000000000000678
2. Barnes JN. Exercise, cognitive function, and aging. *Adv Physiol Educ*. 2015;39(2):55-62. doi:10.1152/advan.00101.2014

3. Carosio S, Berardinelli MG, Aucello M, Musarò A. Impact of ageing on muscle cell regeneration. *Ageing Res Rev*. 2011;10(1):35-42. doi:10.1016/j.arr.2009.08.001

4. Chilton W, O'Brien B, Charchar F. Telomeres, Aging and Exercise: Guilty by Association?. *Int J Mol Sci*. 2017;18(12):2573. Published 2017 Nov 29. doi:10.3390/ijms18122573

5. Cotterell N, Buffel T, Phillipson C. Preventing social isolation in older people. *Maturitas*. 2018;113:80-84. doi:10.1016/j.maturitas.2018.04.014

6. Kivipelto M, Mangialasche F, Ngandu T. Lifestyle interventions to prevent cognitive impairment, dementia and Alzheimer disease. *Nat Rev Neurol*. 2018;14(11):653-666. doi:10.1038/s41582-018-0070-3

7. Mattson MP. Lifelong brain health is a lifelong challenge: from evolutionary principles to empirical evidence. *Ageing Res Rev*. 2015;20:37-45. doi:10.1016/j.arr.2014.12.011

8. Rossman MJ, LaRocca TJ, Martens CR, Seals DR. Healthy lifestyle-based approaches for successful vascular aging. *J Appl Physiol (1985)*. 2018;125(6):1888-1900. doi:10.1152/japplphysiol.00521.2018

9. Steering Committee of the Physicians' Health Study Research Group. Final report on the aspirin component of the ongoing Physicians' Health Study. *N Engl J Med*. 1989;321(3):129-135. doi:10.1056/NEJM198907203210301

10. Siegel AJ, Noakes TD. Aspirin to Prevent Sudden Cardiac Death in Athletes with High Coronary Artery Calcium Scores. *Am J Med*. 2019;132(2):138-141. doi:10.1016/j.amjmed.2018.09.015

11. Siegel AJ. Prerace aspirin to protect susceptible runners

from cardiac arrest during marathons: is opportunity knocking? *Open Heart.* 2015;2(1):e000102. Published 2015 Jul 2. doi:10.1136/openhrt-2014-000102

12. Siegel AJ, Noakes TD. Can pre-race aspirin prevent sudden cardiac death during marathons? *Br J Sports Med.* 2017;51(22):1579-1581. doi:10.1136/bjsports-2016-09691

Chap 11. Don't believe the hype: How to read about health and medicine critically before you change your behavior

The internet, television, newspapers, magazines, books, and advertisements provide an endless stream of new information on diet, nutrition, exercise, health, and medicine. Most of the information is one of the following:

- Presenting a study that seems new and exciting, but is too new to know its' true importance.
- Just repackaging and rehashing old information in a new way.
- Promoting some kind of product that seems to work miracles for "some people" but has little proof behind it.
- A large book with all of the above trying to sell itself.

Even though there are many interesting facts about health, what you really want to know is whether those facts should change your behavior. Human beings have a tendency to think in terms of stories instead of mathematical probabilities. Unfortunately, advertisers and sellers take advantage of this trait when they try to sell you something or convince you to do something their way. Even if something does not work, all they need is one or two good stories to sell it. However, if you want to make truly informed decisions about the information out there, it is important to try to think more objectively, and sometimes statistically. This can apply to almost all the information presented in the news, social media, or the internet. However, I will remain focused on how to properly analyze information related to health, exercise, and diet. If you find new information on a diet or exercise program that claims to make you much healthier, before you change what you do, you have to ask yourself the following:

1. Does the study prove cause and effect, or is it just an interesting association or correlation?
2. Is the study statistically meaningful? Statistics looks at whether a finding is related to a true effect, or whether it can be related to just chance or random luck. I will not go into any details about statistics, but instead will try to provide hypothetical examples of how studies can sometimes be misleading.
3. Does the study apply to you? Even if a study is well designed and statistically solid, it may be looking at a group of people that is very different from you.

Correlation vs Causation?
Should I change my behavior, or is this just an interesting association?

"People who live in Country A drink twice as much wine as Country B, but live much longer."

Does the study show a clear difference between the control group and the treated group, and is that the only difference? Could there be other differences between the two groups that could be the real reason or cause for the results? It is very important to separate cause and effects (causation) from associations (correlation), because true cause and effect findings may convince you to change your behavior. However, if the finding is just a correlation, it is not clear that changing your behavior will have any effect. For example, in the study above, we could not just assume the wine is what makes them live longer. There can be millions of differences between the two countries that could be the real reason for living longer. So it is really hard to say what you should do differently: hopefully you would not use the study as an excuse to drink more wine, because there are many other better designed studies that suggest that alcohol is usually more harmful to health than beneficial.

Is there a placebo effect? What is the control group?
Is the study well designed and honest, or is it biased towards proving something?

"All natural Pep supplement gives people extra energy: people who took Pep supplement twice a day for 4 weeks reported increased energy levels compared to people who didn't take anything."

In this case, the people knew they were taking a supplement for energy, and started to be more aware of when they felt they had higher energy. When asked about their energy levels, they reported higher levels. This was compared to people who took nothing and were not even thinking about their energy levels. The power of suggestion to influence people's behavior and perception, and sometimes even how their body reacts, is an example of the placebo effect.

In the experiment, the study should have compared people who took the pep supplement with people who took a fake pep supplement, without the people knowing if they took the real supplement or the fake one. This is called a blind study, where the subjects do not know whether they are getting a real treatment or a fake one. In addition to the subjects having a bias, it is very possible that the experimenters running the study could have a bias. After all they want to prove their supplement works. So when they interview the patients, the interviewer may unintentionally influence or lead the subjects to give them answers they want to hear. Ideally the interviewers should not even know what group the subject is in. This is known as a double-blind study, where both the subjects in the study and the people measuring the results do not know who is in what group. When the study was redone in a double-blind fashion, they found no difference in energy between the pep supplement and the fake supplement. So clearly, the first study's claim that pep supplement helped energy was not true, but only a placebo effect.

What is being compared?
Does this study really answer the question I am interested in asking? Are there enough details to change my behavior?

"The keto diet leads to an average of 15lbs of weight loss... compared to people on no diet."

"The Atkins diet leads to an average of 15lbs of weight loss... compared to people on no diet."

"An 8 hour intermittent fasting leads to an average of 15 lbs. of weight loss... compared to people on no diet."

"People with Weight Watchers lose an average of 15lb... compared to people without Weight Watchers."

This is the classic way to promote fad diets and interventions that claim to help with weight loss.
Do you see a trend here? Of course, I have exaggerated how similar the results are, but when you put all your studies together you can make one conclusion: "going on some kind of diet can help you lose 15lbs compared to not going on a diet." But the question most people are asking is not "Should I go on a diet." The question most people are asking is "Which diet

should I go on?" None of the studies above answers that question by themselves alone. You have to look at all the studies to conclude that it may not really matter.

Did you ever notice that the commercials or ads promoting a "weight loss" diet rarely claim they are better than another specific "weight loss" diet? That is because the actual kind of diet usually does not make a difference, which means it may be more about being mindful and ultimately cutting portions and calories in some way. Or something else we haven't figured out yet. There is nothing magic about one diet over another. In other words, there were many more differences between the diet and no diet groups than just the type of food itself, or there may be an important aspect of the diet (i.e., total calories) that was not measured or carefully looked at.

"A 1500 calorie high protein diet leads to 15 lbs. more weight loss than a 1500 calorie high fat diet."

In this case, there may be a specific aspect of the high protein diet that needs further investigation, but it still seems to be promising. Clearly it is not just an issue of calories you eat, but there actually seems to be something better about a protein diet over a fat diet for weight loss. Of course, you still have to see what they mean by a high protein diet. Is it all fish? Is it all chicken breast? Can you be sure that a protein diet that is different than the one in the study will lead to the same results? Unless you are willing to adopt the exact same diet detailed in the study, these are the questions you have to ask before changing your behavior.

Can I connect the dots?
"Study after study shows that magnesium is critical for cellular health, protein synthesis, muscle function, nerve

function, blood pressure control, and blood sugar control. If you want to guarantee the best health possible, you need to make sure you are getting enough magnesium every day. Super Mag pills have more usable magnesium than any other on the market..."

The first statement above is true. Our bodies need magnesium for many critical cellular functions. But everything else is just a sophisticated advertisement based on deceptive and false logic. We get more than enough magnesium from the food we eat, even if we are on a low-calorie diet. Magnesium deficiency is extremely rare and tends to occur in people who are chronically malnourished or critically ill. It is something most of us do not need to worry about. Even though you need a small amount of magnesium in your diet to stay healthy, swallowing super doses of magnesium will not make you healthier.

This advertisement goes through the following inferences to convince you to buy their product:

1. Magnesium is critical for cellular health. This is true and proven.
2. Therefore, extra magnesium will improve your health. Not true. And actually, proven to be not true, but they do not share this with you.
3. You might be magnesium deficient. Not true. Extremely unlikely
4. Taking magnesium pills will make you healthier. Once again, not true, and proven to be not true.
5. Super Mag pills have more usable magnesium than others. Maybe true, maybe not. They don't really have a study proving it, but who cares anyway?

The real question you need to ask is:

Is there a study that shows people taking Super Mag pills are actually healthier than people taking other types of magnesium

pills, or people not taking any magnesium at all?
The answer to this would be "Of course not."

How are the numbers presented?
Are the numbers meaningful enough to change my behavior?

"Eating food X TRIPLES the risk of colon cancer in people under age 50!"

Wow, food X sounds deadly.
Numbers and data can be described in many ways. Sometimes articles will present numbers in the most dramatic way possible, to make the study stand out to readers. A common example of this is presenting numbers as increased risk instead of incidence.
In the study above, the incidence of colon cancer in people under age 50 is 8/100,000. This means there are about 8 cases of colon cancer for every 100,000 people. For people under age 50 who eat food X, the incidence of colon cancer is 25 in 100,000. This means that even though eating food X triples the risk, there is still only a very low 0.025% chance of getting colon cancer. So even though the study is well designed and clearly proves an increased risk, is the chance of getting colon cancer high enough that you would avoid food X forever? Food X suddenly does not seem as deadly when presented as incidence instead of risk.

Does the Study have Power?
Does the study look hard enough to make its conclusions true?

The power of a study depends on how many people or subjects the study looks at.

If I gave you a coin that could be either evenly weighted (fair) or weighted to one side, how would you know? You would start flipping to see.

If you got 3 heads out of 3 flips, you might be suspicious that it is weighted for heads, but it is also very possible that the coin is still fair.

If you got 75 heads out of 100 flips, you might once again be suspicious, but still not confident.

If you took the time, and turned up 680,000 heads out of 1,000,000 flips, you might finally start to feel confident that the coin was slightly weighted towards heads.

When a study only looks at a small number of people, there is a greater possibility that the findings and conclusions can also be explained by pure chance. When a study looks at a huge number of people, there is a greater possibility that the findings and conclusions have some truth to them.

"In a double blinded study, supplement X boosted muscle mass compared to a placebo control group, with 0% complications and side effects... based on 200 participants (100 in each group)."

So far, the study above seems promising. The study is designed well, and with only 100 people in each group, they were able to show a clear benefit to using supplement X. Let's say that the actual increase in muscle mass is about 4 pounds. Maybe not that much, but still a clear difference. However, the claim that 0% complications makes it safe is misleading. Whenever a study claims to have a very low complication rate, you have to ask if the study has enough "power" to make that claim. If it turns out that the chance of death from supplement X is actually 1 in 200, would people use it? Absolutely not. For most people, 4 pounds of extra muscle mass would not be worth risking a 1 in 200 chance of death.

There is a very crude formula that says if you study *n* number of patients, and zero patients have a complication, you can be 95% confident that the range of actual complications is somewhere between zero and 3/*n*. In the study above, we can be fairly confident that the chance of having a complication with supplement X is between zero and 3/100, or 3%. This means there still could be a 3 in 100 chance of having a complication. The power of the study using only 100 people to detect complications is still not good enough to call supplement X safe. The only way to know if supplement X is safe is to study more people and keep tracking complications. We have to increase the power. After looking at 10,000 people and seeing 5 complications and 0 deaths, we might feel a little better believing that the supplement is safe.

"In a double blinded study, supplement Y did not boost muscle mass compared to a placebo control group... based on 10 participants in each group."

Based on this study, you might conclude that supplement Y is not worth taking. But once again, whenever a study claims there is NO difference, you have to ask if they looked hard enough. It may turn out that supplement Y does not boost muscle mass by a lot, but it still might boost it by a tiny little bit. When we study supplement Y over groups of a 100 or 1000, we might start to notice the difference. When the number of people studied is small, the power is low, and you will only be able to detect big differences between groups. If the study does not find a difference, it is misleading to say there was no difference. It would be more accurate to say there is no BIG or SUPER OBVIOUS difference. There may still be a small difference that needs more studies to prove or disprove.

"People who successfully lost 15lbs or more on diet X were 10% more likely to have hazel eye color compared to the normal population."

First of all, this study would not affect your behavior in any way, because you cannot really change your eye color. But will your friend with hazel eyes truly be more successful with diet X than someone who has brown eyes? Once again, you have to ask yourself how hard they looked. If they only looked at a small group of people, the finding could be completely random and just pure luck. Just like the coin flip example earlier. You would have to make sure this difference exists after looking at thousands, or perhaps 100's of thousands of people to be confident about it being true.

Are the subjects similar to you?
"A completely plant-based diet increases lifespan by almost 25%... (in mice)"

Experiments in animals such as mice, rats, and other mammals may be extremely well designed, statistically strong, and show great potential. But the overwhelming majority of animal studies will not pan out to be useful to humans. It will be many years before you will know if an animal study actually leads to something useful to humans. A study in cows could show the benefits of eating grass, but clearly that does not apply to you.

"Eating protein shakes BEFORE a workout instead of AFTER increases muscle gain ...in 20 year old men just starting to lift weights 5 days a week."

If the study is done in humans, ask yourself if the subjects are similar to you. If all the people in the studies are the opposite sex, a very different age, or a different race, the results may not apply to you. Did you know people with red hair need more anesthesia? A small fact that shows that even though human beings are essentially the same, there can be small but significant genetic differences that affect how each of us respond to our environment. Certainly sex and age are huge factors in how we respond to different interventions.

Is there a selection bias?
Is there something else about the group we didn't ask?

"Testosterone level in men over age 40 does not seem to correlate with weightlifting... based on blood samples and surveys collected from over 1000 male volunteers ... who learned about the study through flyers posted at multiple gyms."

Selection bias refers to when the group being looked at may not accurately represent the true population. This is very common in any study that looks at a group of "volunteers." Even when volunteers are getting paid, the people who volunteer for scientific studies rarely represent a similar population chosen randomly. If a study is promoted in a specific website or magazine or college campus, then almost all of the volunteers will be people who looked at the promotions. If a study offers $50 for four hours of work, it is probably going to select for people who make less than that or do not work.

"Testosterone level is lower in young men with high bmi compared to young men with normal bmi... based on a retrospective analysis of 200 medical records."

Another example of selection bias usually occurs when the researchers look back through medical records to find correlations. This is called a retrospective study: instead of designing an experiment, recruiting new participants, and trying to control as many variables as possible, researchers simply look for patterns and correlations through data that has already happened in the real world. The study above did not randomly sample young men across the population, but only those young men who had a testosterone level checked. So we need to ask, why did these young men get these levels checked in the first place? Were they having problems with impotence? Were they worried about their inability to gain muscle? Did they read a certain news article? Are some of the participants seeking gender reassignment surgery? Although the study above may have valid findings, we still need to question the selection bias and look for future studies that more accurately represent the real population and that look forward instead of backward.

Are the findings short term or long term?

Is there proof that the effect you see over a short period of time will last over a long period of time?

As I have mentioned many times throughout this book, many fad diets or new exercise plans usually show a successful change over a few weeks or a few months. But we know that it is much harder to maintain these results over years or decades. In the case of diets, many diets show a short-term weight loss in the first few months, but actually lead to more weight gain in the long term when people stop following them. Always look for studies that show sustainability and long-term improvement before you change your behavior.

Even reputable medical journals tend to publish more dramatic results over truer ones.

Studies that show dramatic or interesting results are more likely to get published, even if they don't have enough statistical power. Even in the most prestigious peer reviewed journals, studies that show "boring results" are less likely to get published than more "exciting ones." Suppose we are worried that eggs might increase the chance of heart disease. There may be many studies that show there is no risk with eating eggs a few times a week, but they will not get published in journals because they may not be designed well or have enough power. Suddenly, a study that shows eating seven eggs a week increases the risk of heart disease gets published in a well-respected journal, even though the study also has many flaws. This is because the finding seems too important to ignore. But this is just a bias. Ironically, once the "eggs are bad" study is published, the "eggs are okay" studies suddenly improve their chance of getting published, because now we have an "egg controversy." Eventually, it will take many years and many more studies to settle the matter. And just when you think the matter is settled, suddenly a little flawed study showing that eggs actually decrease heart disease will suddenly get more attention than it deserves.

Beware of anything that sounds like an advertisement:

Beware of supplements and products that cost money, since there is a financial incentive to promote the product. TV and radio shows are full of these well disguised advertisements full of random scientific and medical facts but no actual studies. Even reputable doctors who host these shows eventually compromise and rationalize the products to themselves for the sake of advertising dollars.

Does the headline really describe the conclusions of the study? Articles are written to be read, and just like all news, catchy and dramatic headlines will increase the number of readers. But as you read the study critically, you may realize the headline is a huge oversimplification, and sometimes outright deceptive. Even articles about health and medicine use "clickbait" to increase their views.

Is there a financial or other incentive behind the study? In other words, is this a true study, or is this more of a promotion for a single product or program? Look at who is doing the study, or who is funding the study. Does the product cost money? If the results seem too good to be true, they probably are.

Does the article reference a true study, or is it just a string of anecdotes? If the article makes no mention of experimental design or a control group, it is probably just a series of stories and reviews. These stories are always positive, and there is no way of knowing if there were any negative reviews the authors left out on purpose. This is essentially an advertisement disguised as news.

Conclusion

I am not discouraging you from learning about the latest health and medicine news. In fact, I absolutely encourage it. Overall, it will improve your awareness and understanding of your health in the long term, and that alone will make you a healthier person. I am merely suggesting that you read the news critically, and definitely pause before you let the latest news or study change your behavior.

References

1. Bain BJ, Littlewood TJ, Szydlo RM. The finer points of writing and refereeing scientific articles. *Br J Haematol*. 2016;172(3):350-359. doi:10.1111/bjh.13888
2. Button KS, Ioannidis JP, Mokrysz C, et al. Power failure: why small sample size undermines the reliability of neuroscience [published correction appears in Nat Rev Neurosci. 2013 Jun;14(6):451]. *Nat Rev Neurosci*. 2013;14(5):365-376. doi:10.1038/nrn3475
3. Gardenier JS. Recommendations for describing statistical studies and results in general readership science and engineering journals. *Sci Eng Ethics*. 2012;18(4):651-662. doi:10.1007/s11948-011-9261-7
4. Higginson AD, Munafò MR. Current Incentives for Scientists Lead to Underpowered Studies with Erroneous Conclusions. PLoS Biol. 2016;14(11):e2000995. Published 2016 Nov 10. doi:10.1371/journal.pbio.2000995
5. Prescott RJ, Civil I. Lies, damn lies and statistics: errors and omission in papers submitted to INJURY 2010-2012. *Injury*. 2013;44(1):6-11. doi:10.1016/j.injury.2012.11.005
6. Yasmin, S. Viral BS: Medical Myths and Why We Fall for Them. Johns Hopkins Press. Jan 2021.
7. Zimmer C. How You Should Read Coronavirus Studies, or Any Science Paper
   The New York Times, June 1, 2020.
   https://nyti.ms/3doJ9S3

Chap 12. Random Tips, Adjustments, and Questions

How to choose a gym:

There is no right answer to choose a gym except choose a gym that you are most likely to use. In other words, choose the one that is most convenient. Usually this means choosing one that is close to work or home. Also choose a gym that has power racks for your barbell workouts, and hopefully enough power racks that they are not always being used when you go.

Can I afford a home gym?

Setting up a home gym can be expensive. You can do a fair amount of exercise with the following setup:

Adjustable dumbbells which can range from about $200-$400.

An adjustable inclined bench which can be purchased for $150 - $200.

A doorway pull-up bar for under $100.

For aerobic activity, if you cannot run or bike outside due to the weather, you can consider an inexpensive spin bike which can range from $200 to $300, or a trainer for your regular bike which can be less than $100. Treadmills and Stairmasters are more expensive.

Of course, everything can be found cheaper if bought used instead of new.

Weight etiquette and tips:

When using a power rack or bench, do not walk away too long. If you are going to walk away, leave something there (your water bottle, keys, etc.) so people know you are not done. When you are done, remove all the weights from the bar, and stack weights and dumbbells back onto the rack. If you used a bench, wipe it off.

How much does the barbell bar weigh?

The barbells used for squats and deadlift are usually Olympic barbells with 2-inch diameter ends. These are supposed to weigh 45lbs. So, if you bench press the bar with two 45lb plates, you are lifting around 45 + 45 + 45 = 135 lbs.

How to improve grip strength:

When using the barbell and dumbbells, use some powder or talc to improve your grip and prevent slipping. You can try weight gloves if they help, but most people do not find they help that much. Sometimes they widen the diameter of your grip, making your grip weaker. Exercises that improve grip strength include the deadlift, pull ups, just hanging by a bar, or the farmer's walk exercise (walk straight carrying heavy dumbbells for a short distance).

How to adjust if one side is much stronger than the other:

Use your weaker non dominant side to carry and stack weights between your sets. You may want to consider focusing more on the dumbbell exercises which require you to work on each side independently.

How to adjust when not getting stronger:

Here are some things to try if you feel that you have not gotten stronger for many months but still feel you have potential for improvement.

- Whenever you have some extra time, add in additional weight exercises on your weakest muscles. If your legs are making no progress, add in more leg exercises. Or if you feel pretty good about your strength in one muscle group, skip it for a few weeks or even months and spend the extra time on your weaker muscle groups.

- During every exercise, pay attention to your weakest muscle, and try to incorporate more exercises into your routine that strengthen that particular weakness. For example, if you find that your deadlift is being limited by your grip rather than your back, try to make sure you do exercises that increase grip strength with your workouts. This can include more deadlift, pull ups, and some forearm exercises.
- Drop your weight and focus on form. Having a heavy weight may make you feel stronger, but if you are sacrificing form, you are not working your muscle maximally with each exercise. Ignore what other people around you are lifting. Choose a weight that you can lift slowly and with good form. Increase your frequency to 10 to 12 with each rep, but still choose a high enough weight that makes the last reps a struggle.
- Consider resting longer between sets if your strength is dropping off too much between sets.
- Try changing your reps and weights to make your workout more interesting. If you are consistently lifting at 10 reps, try lightening the weight and aiming for 12 to 16. Or try increasing the weight and aiming for just 4 to 6. Or, if you have enough time between each set to change the weight, try a pyramid set where you keep increasing the weight with each set until you can only do 4 to 6. Ultimately any variation is okay, and usually enough change to kickstart some improvement.
- Sometimes taking a rest week or two without any weights at all will allow you to return with more focus and determination.
- Make sure you are getting enough protein every day.

Is it okay to swap the exercises between workout 1 and workout 2?

Yes, there is no reason you have to do all the barbell or all the dumbbell exercises on one day. You may want to swap some of the exercises between workout 1 and 2 as long as they involve the same muscle group. In other words, try to do at least one leg, back, chest, and preferably shoulder for each workout. And try to do at least one heavy weight (barbell or dumbbell) exercise for each group at least once a week. For example, you may choose to do the barbell squat, the barbell deadlift on workout 1, but save the barbell bench press for workout 2.

Using supersets and alternating exercises to save time.

There is a lot of hype about supersets (or compound exercises), which involve doing multiple sets of different exercises without rest between sets.

If the exercises primarily work the same muscle group (i.e., all biceps or all shoulders) the science suggests that supersets do not help and most likely lead to fatigue and muscle damage without any benefit to growth. In addition, you can only pick the weight based on your weakest muscle group. Therefore, they don't provide much advantage considering they take longer to do.

On the other hand, you can shorten your rest time between sets if you alternate your sets between opposing muscle groups (agonist-antagonist). An example of this is doing one set of triceps immediately followed by one set of biceps. You do not require as much rest between each set when you do this, which can shorten your overall time in the gym. If you decide to not rest at all, and create a superset with opposing muscle groups, there actually may be some benefit. The reasons for this are unclear, but it is possible that stretching the opposing muscle while contracting a muscle may help promote growth.

The biggest disadvantage to alternating muscle groups is that you need two sets ups. It probably does not make sense for the barbell heavy weight exercises, which would require you to have two power cages and two barbells. In addition, most of these exercises need your full strength, which means you probably need to rest as long as possible. It's easier to do some of the dumbbell exercises as alternating sets with minimal or no rest. You can do back alternating with chest or triceps alternating with biceps. If you are up to it, it's definitely another way to save time.

Ref: Brentano MA, Umpierre D, Santos LP, et al. Muscle Damage and Muscle Activity Induced by Strength Training Super-Sets in Physically Active Men. *J Strength Cond Res.* 2017;31(7):1847-1858. doi:10.1519/JSC.0000000000001511

Isn't this a strength training routine rather than a muscle size building routine?

If you are asking this question, you have probably done some investigation into various programs and found lots of discussion debating programs that develop strength vs programs that develop muscle size. In simplest terms, programs that focus on higher weights and less repetition are thought to promote strength, while those that focus on less weight but much more repetition can lead to larger muscle size. Based on that generalization, this program is probably prioritizing developing strength over muscle size. However, this distinction really applies to advanced weightlifters who are deciding to become competitive weightlifters vs competitive bodybuilders. For beginners and intermediate lifters, the difference is irrelevant. This program will increase your strength and increase your muscle size while keeping the workouts as short and efficient as possible. Ultimately, I would argue that, especially for older men, functional strength is much more important than looking big. It allows you to be more active in all aspects of your life while avoiding injury. (Your partner will also find your strength to be more useful around the house moving furniture, lifting packages, and carrying heavy groceries).

Can the program in this book be used for women?

Most of the concepts described in this book will apply to women as well as men. As far as we know, the mechanisms of muscle formation and fat loss are essentially the same. All the dietary recommendations are identical for women as well. The body fat percentage chart for women is different, and the waist size threshold for women is different. As mentioned before, for women, a waist size of 42 inches has twice the risk of death compared to a waist size of 29.5 inches or less. The risks of heart disease and diabetes start to increase over 40 inches for men and 35 inches for women.

There are more hormonal factors that can affect the way women respond to exercise and diet, and I did not address the studies on that in this book. The responses to the interventions in this book can be more variable in women than men. In addition, there are more body types in women compared to men. Specifically, there are some women who have relatively normal waists but more fat in their bottoms and thighs, and even though this type of fat may not increase the risk of disease, they may want to still reduce this fat for cosmetic reasons.

Although I do believe much of the information in this book is applicable to women, I did not gear this book towards women because I feel there is additional information applicable to women that I did not include.

Can I use protein shakes as a meal replacement if I am trying to lose fat?

The answer is yes if it works for you and is satisfying enough to work as a replacement. In general, it is not something you can do lifelong, but if you find it helpful in losing fat, there is probably no harm in trying it. It helps some people and not others. The most important thing to remember is that if you stop using it as a meal replacement, keep a close eye on your weight every day so you don't start gaining again. This is something you should be doing anyway.

Is stretching important?

There are three types of stretching.

1. Static stretching is the act of stretching out a muscle to its full extension and holding it as long as possible. There is very little movement. This is what most think of when we think of stretching.
2. Dynamic stretching is moving a limb through its full range of motion several times. There is a lot of movement.
3. Pre-contraction stretching includes a variety of exercises where the muscle is contracted for several seconds before being stretched. These are more like exercises, and they are often used and taught by physical therapists.

There is a LOT of research on stretching, and there are many contradictory studies. However, for the most part, when all the studies are combined, most experts on the subject make the following recommendations:

- Developing flexibility of the hips and legs is functionally more important than flexibility in the torso, upper body, or neck. To increase flexibility and range of motion, all the types of stretching can be used. Static stretching is recommended for the elderly.

- For strength and performance, static stretching prior to exercise or playing a sport can actually decrease performance (unless it is for gymnastics, dancing, or a sport that requires flexibility during the sport). For this reason, static stretching is not recommended before exercise and most sports (i.e., running, biking, basketball, etc.). Instead, dynamic stretching should be used to warm up before exercise or competition.
- Stretching before or after exercise probably does not prevent injury.

Reference:
Page P. Current concepts in muscle stretching for exercise and rehabilitation. *Int J Sports Phys Ther.* 2012;7(1):109-119.

How do I deal with pain or injury?

Ultimately, you must use good judgement whenever you have pain or injury, and you should avoid anything that can make it worse. When you do resistance exercises involving a susceptible joint, make sure to use proper form and do not try to use weights too high to maintain good form.

If you have a short-term injury like a sprain or ligament inflammation, do not do any exercise that makes it hurt more, and make sure it is completely healed for a few weeks before starting an exercise that might flare it up again. When you restart, start with very low weights and always use good form. For arm inflammation such as tennis elbow or tendinitis, try to change the grip of your exercises to prevent re-inflammation. If you have shoulder pain, try a shoulder exercise that does not reproduce the pain. This might mean not lifting above your head or lifting your arms in front of you rather than the side. Sometimes elbow and forearm pain is often worse with arm exercises like biceps and triceps exercises but does not flare up with chest or back exercises.

If you have long term or recurring injuries like back pain or hip pain or knee pain, once again pay attention to any exercise that makes it worse, and always maintain good form rather than trying to lift too much weight.

Needless to say, if you are unsure about how to exercise around your injury, consult with a qualified sports medicine doctor or a physical therapist.

In the long term, a regular resistance exercise routine will prevent joint injury by strengthening the muscles around your joints, improving your posture, and improving your strength.

What if I want to train for a race?

The workout described is the MINIMUM workout the average man needs to do to stay strong, healthy, look decent, and live longer. At some point, you may want to consider signing up for a competition or race: a 5K, 10K, half marathon, marathon, triathlon, tough mudder, a spartan race, or something similar. Should you do it? Absolutely. If you can, it's a great experience and will give you incentive to push yourself even further. If you want to be confident about doing your best, you should prepare and train for at least a few months before. And it will require more training and time on top of what I have described so far. That being said, if you have been doing this program for a while and feel like you are finally in reasonable shape, you can put this program on hold for a few months to focus on race specific training. After your race, because of muscle memory, you will be able to make up for any lost strength pretty quickly. Each race requires a different skillset. For example, a triathlon may require you to focus on your freestyle open water swim, and a Spartan may require you to climb a rope, run up hills, and swing from monkey bars. (And of course, get very good at burpees). You will have to turn to the internet and other sources on the best way to improve your race specific skills prior to race. I personally have put my weight plan on hold for several months prior to a triathlon to focus on my swimming and running. Most of the time I lost very little muscle and was able to lift with my prior strength within a few weeks.

Should I take vitamins?

Most men do not need to take vitamin supplements unless they are on an extremely low-calorie diet (i.e., less than 1000 calories a day) or have a known vitamin deficiency based on an underlying disease or bloodwork.

So far there are no proven huge benefits to long term multivitamin use in men. There may be a small reduction in cancer risk and some other rare conditions, but otherwise no significant benefit. On the other hand, there are no real risks either as long as you do not take high doses of individual vitamins. Stick with just the generic multivitamins. So, if you do not mind spending the money and taking a large pill every day, you can. But if that seems like an inconvenience, you are okay not taking one as well.

Women are more prone to anemia, osteoporosis, and also B deficiencies during pregnancy. Therefore, women should consult with their doctors and gynecologists regularly about whether they should take supplements or not, since the recommendations are continually changing.

Should I take creatine?

I will not go into the many studies that detail the benefits of creatine. Overall, it seems to be a safe supplement for most people. It definitely does lead to increased water content in muscles and does seem to help most weightlifters build muscle faster. I do not really talk about it or recommend it in this book for the following reasons:

- There are no health benefits to taking it. It is strictly for helping with muscle growth.

- Although it may help with muscle growth, most of the studies are done in people who lift weights much more than twice a week. So, it is difficult to assume it will still be beneficial if you are only lifting twice a week.
- Creatine needs to be taken daily to be effective. It tastes bad, can upset your stomach, and does cost money. I cannot imagine someone wanting to take creatine for the rest of their lives.
- Creatine is helpful for building muscle and traditional "bulking", but it also increases water content in the skin, making you look a bit fatter even though it is actually water and not fat. So it can actually make the muscles look less defined.

Chap 13. A Quick Summary and Request

By now, you have probably figured out that the aim of this book is not to give you a detailed program that is guaranteed to succeed forever. Instead, the goal is to give you a starting point and the skills to modify it into an individualized program that works for your specific body and your lifestyle. You may end up doing completely different exercises than the ones I recommend, and you may ultimately choose a very different diet than the one I recommend. That is fine, as long as it works for you, you feel healthier and happier, and you are able to maintain your program lifelong.

Yes, in the end it is all about diet and exercise. However, hopefully by now you feel that diet and exercise is not as hard as it sounds when done in an efficient, thoughtful way.

The main points of the book can be simplified into the following concepts:

1. MEASURE. Measure your exercise, measure your diet, measure your movement, and measure your progress. If you tend to gain weight easily, measure your weight several times a week no matter what you are doing.
2. RESISTANCE TRAIN 2-3x/week. Resistance training builds muscle, which promotes better long-term function, resilience, and health.
   a. Big muscles (legs, back, chest, shoulders) should be worked out 2 times a week. Never more than 3 times a week.
   b. Other muscles (arms, calves, abdominals) can be worked out 0 - 2 times a week.
3. AEROBIC TRAIN 2-7x/wk. Aerobic training improves

cardiovascular fitness. HITT activities can be shorter (i.e., 10 minutes) while steady pace activities may require more time (20-30 minutes). Do some type of aerobic activity a minimum of twice a week. There is no maximum.

4. MOVE ALL DAY. Movement throughout the day helps maintain weight, improves posture, and prevents injury.
5. EAT HEALTHY 80% of the time. Count calories and increase calories a small amount to gain muscle and decrease calories a small amount to lose fat. Choose protein, avoid sugar. Drink water, avoid alcohol. Avoid eating in the late evening.
6. AVOID ADDICTION: Don't smoke cigarettes, don't vape, don't chew tobacco, don't get addicted to other drugs, substances, or vices.

If I had to choose just one word to describe the key to staying healthy for the rest of your life, I would choose this one:

AWARENESS

Stay aware on a daily basis. If you maintain your awareness, you will use the tools you have learned to stay healthy.

I have used these recommendations in a variety of forms for myself, my patients, my family, and my friends. When followed they work very well. I would greatly appreciate comments and feedback on how well these recommendations have worked for you, and what modifications or changes you would make. Ultimately, I learned more from my patients than they did from me, and I would appreciate a chance to learn from your experience as well so I can continue to improve upon my recommendations.

Promotion and marketing and social media are not my strengths.
So, if you have found this book useful, and worth the small investment, please recommend it to someone you know.

Would love to hear your comments, feedback, and your own modifications on
Amazon   or   Facebook (www.facebook.com/getstronglifelong)

Worksheets are posted on the Facebook site
When writing a review, please let me know how long you were able to keep your routine up. My goal is to come up with something that will last for you.

Wishing you a long and healthy life!

About the author

Sanjoy Dutta, M.D. is a graduate of Yale University and Harvard Medical School. He completed his surgical and research training at the University of California, San Francisco, and has been a practicing general and bariatric (weight loss) surgeon for the past 15 years. During this time, he has been involved in medical research and publications, and has counseled thousands of patients on weight loss and health.

During his free time he enjoys writing, drawing, exercising, and occasionally participating in sprint triathlons. He currently lives in Northern California with his wonderful wife, daughters, and two dogs. He is immensely grateful to live in a world where you can be 50 years old and appreciate life more than ever.

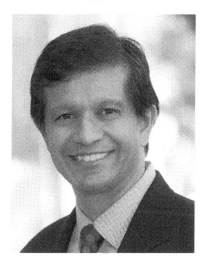

Printed in Great Britain
by Amazon

60109705R00131